MENTAL SURVIVAL GUIDE

COVID-19
EDITION

MENTAL SURVIVAL GUIDE COVID-19

EDITION

The Mental Health Guide for the COVID-19 pandemic

Regain your sanity and relationships while decreasing anxiety, depression, and conflicts

Todd Huston M.A.
Julie Dunbar, LMSW

Host of Love Leaders Podcast

"Eliminate the fear in your mind and the danger in your world."

ISBN 978-0-9980754-5-7

Copyright © 2020 by Todd Huston M.A.

All rights reserved by the copyright holder. No part of this book may be used or reproduced in any form or by any electronic or mechanical means, including information storage and retrieval systems, without permission in writing from the author.

www.ToddHuston.com

Disclaimer: The contents of in the Survival Manual for COVID-19, such as text, graphics, images, and other material contained are for informational purposes only. All information is provided "as is" and there are no representations or warranties of any kind with respect to the book's contents. There are no promises or guarantees being stated in the information or for any results. Any references to other published works in the book are for convenience only and no warranties or representation to the accuracy of the information. The content is not intended to be a substitute for professional advice, diagnosis, or treatment. Always seek the advice of your mental health professional or other qualified health provider with any questions you may have regarding your condition.

If you are in crisis or you think you may have an emergency, call your doctor or 911 immediately. If you are having suicidal thoughts, call the National Suicide Prevention Lifeline at 1-800-273-TALK (8255) to talk to a skilled, trained counselor at a crisis center in your area at any time. If you are located outside the United States, call your local emergency line immediately.

PRINTED IN THE UNITED STATES OF AMERICA

*Dedicated to my wonderful sons, Josh and Zach,
and to my loving wife Julie.*

Life is a lesson in love.

— Todd Huston, M.A.

INTRODUCTION

We are in an unprecedented time. The COVID-19 pandemic has affected most everyone on the planet, and each person handles it differently. For some it is an inconvenience, but for others it takes them to the edge with fear, anxiety, and major depression. This course has easy to understand lessons that will help you now.

According to a study by San Diego University and Florida State University, mental health distress and illness rose over 700 percent after the COVID-19 pandemic began. Considering stress reportedly causes over 90 percent of first visits to primary care physicians, you can't ignore stress if you want to be healthy.

Holocaust survivor and psychiatrist Victor Frankl said, "Forces beyond your control can take away everything you possess except one thing: your freedom to choose how you will respond to the situation." Each individual's situation is unique during this COVID-19 pandemic. Some have lost their jobs and income. Others have retained their jobs or have money in the bank, but have pre-existing physical or mental health conditions, or are elderly. Some have friends and family to support them, while others are isolated and lonely. Again, everyone's situation is different. However, we all have that freedom to choose how we will respond. Each person has the power to think and act on their own behalf and turn a challenging condition into a learning experience that makes them stronger, wiser, and healthier. I know this book will help you along this path. You are not alone. We are taking this journey together.

You are what you think. Unfortunately, external sources, such as the media, have learned to play on our emotions to manipulate our thoughts. For example, some news and media outlets bank on creating fear to trigger our survival instinct, which in turn makes us feel as though we must keep watching their programs to gain the knowledge we hope will help us feel safe again. It's a vicious cycle.

Another challenge we face is dealing with our own irrational thoughts, which can make times like this even more difficult. Science has returned to the idea that mind and body are not separated. Therefore, our thoughts about ourselves not only affect how we deal with others throughout the day, they also affect us physically. This is seen in studies such as the negative effects of mental stress on physical health.

Welcome to the world where your thoughts affect your happiness and health. The COVID-19 pandemic has triggered within many stressors that have lain dormant until now. This workbook will help you understand and modify the thinking and behaviors that generated these stressors, and we will work together to create a healthier you.

I initially wrote this course for a 10,000-employee hospital, for their patients, physicians, and health care staff. It was also used for mental health patients, executive retreats, and at Fortune 500 companies as a workbook and seminar. This edition has modifications to deal specifically with the COVID-19 pandemic, which has created fear and stress for many, and I hope the information will help those who are finding difficulty coping with it. When the pandemic passes and the world is back to normal there will still be stress, so this course will still be valuable to you. I used the best information available about stress and condensed it into short, easy to understand lessons that take only a few minutes to learn.

I hope you enjoy your journey as you learn how to create a better reality through your thoughts and actions. At the end of this course you will be able to recognize the stressors in your life and minimize or eliminate them. Enjoy life, and love often and everywhere.

Life is a lesson in love,
Todd Huston, M.A.

COVID-19 MENTAL SURVIVAL GUIDE

LESSON OUTLINE

This book has 44 Lessons.
Each lesson is divided into four easy to read parts.

Part 1. A Quote: An inspirational quote and a humorous quote or saying.

Part 2. Something to Learn: Knowledge – Information to help you understand stress.

Part 3. Something to Do: Stress Management Tool – A technique to reduce your stress.

Part 4. Something to Write: Journal Entry – A place to record your life and thoughts.

You will see from the Table of Contents that I also divided the book into 3 Sections. Section I will help you learn about and identify stress in your body. Sometimes people don't realize their physical symptoms are stress related. This section helps with that. Section II covers common stressors people experience, from work to home and relationships. Section III focuses on how to manage stress. Each section has valuable information to help you reduce stress.

Note. You do not need to use every technique in this book to reduce your stress. Feel free to find some stress reduction techniques that work best for you and practice using them. The more you use them the more effective they become.

Above all, enjoy doing them!

TODD HUSTON

COVID-19 MENTAL SURVIVAL GUIDE

TABLE OF CONTENTS

Info from the Center for Disease Control (CDC) 10

Section I: Recognizing Stress in the Body and Mind

Lesson 1: History of Stress 17

Lesson 2: Definitions of Stress 21

Lesson 3: Types of Stress 25

Lesson 4: The Body and Stress 29

Lesson 5: Stress Predictors 33

Lesson 6: The "Fight, Flight, or Freeze" Response 37

Lesson 7: Health and Stress 41

Lesson 8: The Mind and Stress 45

Lesson 9: Emotions and Stress 49

Lesson 10: Signs that your Mind is Stressed 53

Lesson 11: Perceptions and Attitudes 57

Lesson 12: Values and Goals 61

Section II: Life's Common Stressors

Lesson 13: Time and Stress 65

Lesson 14: Pareto Principle (80/20 Rule) 69

Lesson 15: Procrastination 73

Lesson 16: Financial Stress 77

Lesson 17: Organizational Stress 81

Lesson 18: Work Stress 85

Lesson 19: Work from Home 89

Lesson 20: Anger and Stress 93

Lesson 21: Couple's Stress 97

Lesson 22: Parenting Stress 101

Lesson 23: Relationship Stress 105

Lesson 24: Caregiver Stress – Compassion Fatigue 109

Section III: Managing Stress

Lesson 25: The ABC's of Stress Management 113

Lesson 26: De-Stress Engineering 117

Lesson 27: Survival Strategies for Life-Threatening Stressors 121

Lesson 28: Physical Activity 125

Lesson 29: Sleep and Stress 129

Lesson 30: Sense of Touch and Stress 133

Lesson 31: Sense of Sight and Stress 137

Lesson 32: Sense of Taste and Stress 141

Lesson 33: Sense of Smell and Stress 145

Lesson 34: Sense of Hearing and Stress 149

Lesson 35: Mindfulness 153

Lesson 36: Mental Imagery and Visualization 157

Lesson 37: Resilience 161

Lesson 38: Social Support 165

Lesson 39 Humor 169

Lesson 40 Forgiveness 173

Lesson 41 Gratitude 177

Lesson 42 Love 181

Lesson 43 Spirituality 185

Lesson 44 Maintaining Your Stress-Resilient Life 189

Appendix

Logs: Anger, Goals Setting, Sleep, Time Management .... 192 - 196

Stress Test and Symptom 201

Values List 207

Common Thought Distortions 210

Resources for Mental Help Assistance
During COVID-19 Pandemic (USA) 215

Table of Contents for Stress Management Tools

To help you find specific stress tools within the Lessons that work well for you.

Stress Tool 1: The Relaxation Response 18

Stress Tool 2: Value of Stress Reduction 22

Stress Tool 3: Goals for Reducing Stress 26

Stress Tool 4: One Minute Body Scan 30

Stress Tool 5: Autogenic Training 34

Stress Tool 6: Diaphragmatic Breathing 38

Stress Tool 7: Hand on Belly Breathing 42

Stress Tool 8: Alternate Nostril Breathing.....................................46

Stress Tool 9: Know Your Emotions..50

Stress Tool 10: Complete Breathing (Zen Breathing) 54

Stress Tool 11: Guided Imagery...58

Stress Tool 12: Guided Imagery II 62

Stress Tool 13: Urgent/Important Principle 66

Stress Tool 14: Using the Pareto Principle.....................................70

Stress Tool 15: Stop Procrastinating..74

Stress Tool 16: Create a Budget 78

Stress Tool 17: Steps to Getting Organized 82

Stress Tool 18: Making SMART Goals 86

Stress Tool 19: Work/Time Routine 90

Stress Tool 20: Meditation..94

Stress Tool 21: Active Listening 98

Stress Tool 22: Parent Communication.......................................102

Stress Tool 23: Quick Calming Techniques.................................106

Stress Tool 24: Avoiding Caregiver Burnout 110

Stress Tool 25: Thought Stopping 114

Stress Tool 26: Solution Focused Visualization 118

Stress Tool 27: Fear vs. Danger 122

Stress Tool 28: Exercise to Reduce Stress 126

Stress Tool 29: Dream Therapy 130

Stress Tool 30: Touch and Relax 134

Stress Tool 31: Color Therapy 138

Stress Tool 32: Eat Away Stress 142

Stress Tool 33: Aromatherapy 146

Stress Tool 34: Nature's Sights and Sounds Therapy 150

Stress Tool 35: Mindfulness Meditation 154

Stress Tool 36: Visualization 158

Stress Tool 37: Building Resilience 162

Stress Tool 38: Support Therapy 166

Lesson 39 Laugh Away Your Stress 170

Lesson 40 Nine Steps to Forgiveness 174

Lesson 41 Gratitude in Action 178

Lesson 42 Life is a Lesson in Love 182

Lesson 43 Prayer 186

Lesson 44 Relaxation Reminders 190

TODD HUSTON

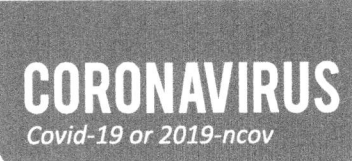
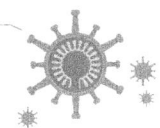

CORONAVIRUS
Covid-19 or 2019-ncov

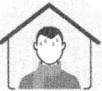
Stay at home
When sick

Avoid close contact
With sick person

Wash your hands
At least 20 seconds

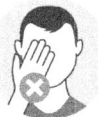
Dont touch your eyes,
nose, & mouth with
Unwashed hand

Clean & disinfect
frequently touched
object & surfaces

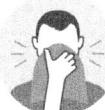
Cover your cough
or sneeze with
a tissue

Don't eat raw food,
throughly cook
meat & eggs

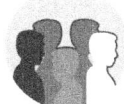
Avoid Crowd
Places

 ## SYMPTOMS

Common

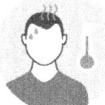
Fever

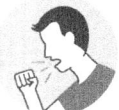
Dry cough

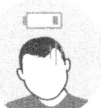
Fatigue

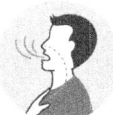
Shortness of
Breath

Less typical

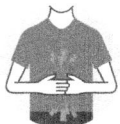
Diarrhea

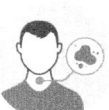
Phelgm buildup

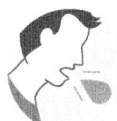
Hemoptysis

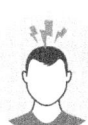
Headache

TRANSMISSION

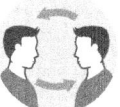
Person-to-person

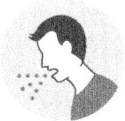
Respiratory droplets
Of infected person

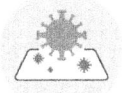
Touching a surface
where virus landed
recently

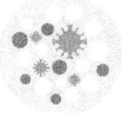
Aerosol

Info from the Center for Disease Control (CDC)

COVID-19 and Stress

The outbreak of Coronavirus disease 2019 (COVID-19) may be stressful for people. Fear and anxiety about a disease can be overwhelming and cause strong emotions in adults and children. Coping with stress will make you, the people you care about, and your community stronger.

Stress during an infectious disease outbreak can include

- Fear and worry about your own health and the health of your loved ones
- Changes in sleep or eating patterns
- Difficulty sleeping or concentrating
- Worsening of chronic health problems
- Worsening of mental health conditions
- Increased use of alcohol, tobacco, or other drugs

Everyone reacts differently to stressful situations

How you respond to the outbreak can depend on your background, the things that make you different from other people, and the community you live in.

People who may respond more strongly to the stress of a crisis include

- Older people and people with chronic diseases who are at higher risk for severe illness from COVID-19
- Children and teens
- People who are helping with the response to COVID-19, like doctors, other health care providers, and first responders
- People who have mental health conditions including problems with substance use

What You Need to Know Now:

Stress During the Pandemic

The safer you feel, the less stress you will experience during the COVID-19 pandemic. When you take care of your physical needs for protection and survival, you will make your environment safer for you and for others. Always practice good hygiene, have plenty of food and supplies, and continue to socialize while practicing social distancing. Try to retain as much normalcy as possible without putting yourself or others at risk. The less you are exposed to danger, the safer and less stressed you will feel.

Practice hygiene

- Wash hands frequently with soap and water for at least 20 seconds or use hand sanitizer.
- Cover your mouth and nose with a tissue when you cough or sneeze.
- Social distance 6-9 feet (2-3 meters) apart from others.
- Limit non-essential travel and shopping.
- Avoid touching your face.
- Wash clothes and bedding.
- Cough or sneeze into your upper sleeve, arm, or elbow if you don't have a tissue.
- Clean your hands after coughing or sneezing. Properly dispose of used tissues.
- Stay at home if you are sick and self-quarantine. Wear a mask to not expose others.
- Avoid contact with those who are sick. Wear a mask and gloves when needed.
- Clean and disinfect objects or surfaces that may have come into contact with germs.
- Make plans for what will happen if someone in the home becomes ill or if quarantine or shelter-in-place measures are ordered.

Practice Self Care

- Keep your body and mind active – do puzzles, read, have a to-do list, exercise.
- Sleep and have time to relax, create a routine, try mindfulness apps.
- Stay informed at CDC.gov.
- Eat healthy and stay hydrated – avoid excess caffeine and alcohol.
- Bathe and groom.
- Limit exposure to social media and negative news, especially before bedtime.
- Stay socially connected with phone calls, email, social media, text, and video chat.
- Try to be helpful to others.
- Practice your spiritual beliefs – listen and read the works of those who inspire you.

Have Supplies

- Water and food, vitamins, fluids with electrolytes, and food preparation items.
- Prescribed medical supplies or equipment, such as glucose or blood pressure monitoring equipment; thermometer; medicines for fever, anti-diarrheal medication.
- Hygiene supplies such as soap and water, alcohol-based hand wash, soap, tissues, toilet paper, and disposable diapers if necessary.
- General supplies such as a flashlight and batteries, portable radio, and garbage bags.
- Be prepared, but you don't need to be a hoarder. This pandemic will pass.

Although anyone may experience increased anxiety at this time, the CDC has identified those who may be at increased risk:

- Older adults and those with chronic diseases
- Children and teens

- People helping with the response to COVID-19, such as healthcare providers, first responders, grocery store workers, and custodial staff
- In a cross-sectional survey, many Chinese healthcare workers reported symptoms of depression (50.4%), anxiety (44.6%), insomnia (34.0%), and distress (71.5%) during the COVID-19 outbreak.
- People who have mental health conditions including problems with substance use including alcohol

JOURNAL ENTRY Tips

Journaling helps you get the thoughts out of your head by writing them down so you can be clearer and more focused. There are no right or wrong journal entries! It's just about your thoughts on paper. Here are seven steps to effective JOURNAL ENTRY that will help you as you go through the lessons in this book.

1. **Centering**. Take a moment to relax before writing.

2. **Labeling.** Record day, date, and year of each entry.

3. **Uncensored.** Write whatever comes to your mind. Ignore grammar and neatness.

4. **Spontaneity.** Write, draw, or compose poetry or song.

5. **Freedom.** Express your thoughts freely.

6. **Get comfy**. Identify indoor and outdoor places where you feel comfortable journaling.

8. **Privacy.** Keep your JOURNAL ENTRY to yourself. Be discreet if you share.

9. **Writer's block**. Start with a question. Don't fear what may come out of you.

TODD HUSTON

*Just when the caterpillar thought the world was ending,
she became a butterfly.*

- Barbara Haines Howett

If they would have posted this on Facebook
as the Stay at home challenge,
the virus would be gone by now.

LESSON 1
LESSON: History of Stress

You need the stress response to survive. Our ancestors had to worry about lions, tigers, and warring tribes, so they needed the stress response to cheat death on a daily basis. Though we likely won't find ourselves wiping the sweat from our brow after outsmarting a tiger, we have stressors just as challenging today. We may face a thief breaking into our home or a car that ran a red light and is coming right at us, making this hardwired response necessary for our survival.

Today the COVID-19 pandemic has definitely generated this response. The fear of contracting the disease, being quarantined, social-distancing, home schooling, job disruptions, loss of income, and many other issues have created a mental health firestorm. Add it to our normal stressors of deadlines, arguments with a co-worker or spouse, financial struggles, road rage, out-of-control children, a public speaking engagement, or meeting someone new, and it's no surprise we feel the wear and tear on our bodies and minds.

Fortunately, we now know how to manage and cope with stress.

EXERCISE:
The Relaxation Response

The Relaxation Response is a powerfully built-in healing mechanism for rest and recovery from stressful events. Without it we may unwittingly choose a fight, flight, or freeze response. The Relaxation Response consists of a natural set of physiological changes that offset the stress response, including:

- Heart rate slows down
- Breathing declines
- Blood pressure decreases
- Body metabolism lowers
- Muscles relax

Observe your heart rate and breathing. Is your heart racing, or normal? Is your breathing fast and shallow, or deep and slow? Are your muscles tense, or relaxed? If your muscles are tense, where do you feel it? In your neck, shoulders, or somewhere else?

Take time to notice how your body reacts to stress and how you feel when you are not stressed so you will know when and how stress affects you.

JOURNAL ENTRY

What stressful events do you hope to minimize or eliminate in your life now?

How will your life be different with reduced stress?

The eagle does not escape the storm.
The eagle simply uses the storm to lift it higher. It spreads its
mighty wings and rises on the winds that bring the storm.

- Jack White

Due to the increase in home deliveries,
FEDx and UPS have merged
and become FED-UP.

LESSON 2
LESSON: Definitions of Stress

Stress is the wear and tear brought on by perceived threats and coping deficiencies. Put simply, if you are in a situation you think threatens your health, well-being, needs, or wants – and you think there's little you can do about it – you have the basic ingredients for stress.

Stress is a change in your physical, mental, or emotional state. It is brought about by a real or perceived stressor, which can be external or internal.

Stressful wear and tear can be detrimental to your physical and mental health. Your thoughts about the COVID-19 pandemic may be causing stress, or wear and tear, on your body and mind. This can cause you to feel frustrated, angry, depressed, have lower levels of energy, or other stress-related symptoms.

Coping and managing stress is when you recognize a potential stressor, or that you are experiencing stress, and you take action to minimize or eliminate it. This is also called stress reduction, and is the purpose of the lessons in this book.

EXERCISE:
Value of Stress Reduction

What do you hope to accomplish by having less stress? Look at the list below and mark any of the benefits of stress reduction you would appreciate. If you don't see something, add it to the list.

- Reduces anxiety, fear, and panic
- Decreases chronic tension and chronic diseases like diabetes
- Decreases pain and need for pain medications
- Reduces blood pressure
- Decreases risk of heart disease
- Improves comfort during medical, surgical, and dental procedures
- Reduces the length of labor and discomfort of childbirth
- Lessens the stress of infertility and improves the chances of conception
- Speeds healing and recovery from surgery, injury, or skin problems
- Boosts the immune function
- Eases sleep problems
- Makes you look and feel younger

JOURNAL ENTRY

List your top five stressors during the past three months, or during the COVID-19 pandemic, and how they affected you. These can include job, children, relationships, financial, or any other areas of stress in your life. How does stress feel for you? Do you get irritable, do your muscles tighten, or do you have headaches? Write about it.

1.

2.

3.

4.

5.

TODD HUSTON

*The last human freedom is to choose
one's attitude in any given situation.*

- Viktor Frankl

Now I know how my dog feels.
I roam the house for food.
I am told not to get close to strangers
and I look forward to getting out for a walk
or ride in the car.

LESSON 3
LESSON: Types of Stress

Eustress. Stress that comes from positive and constructive experiences, like marriage, the birth of child, Christmas and holidays, vacations, or a new relationship. Positive stress adds anticipation and excitement to life, and we thrive under a certain amount of it.

Neustress. Neutral stress. When events have neither a good nor a bad effect.

Distress. This is what most people refer to when they say they are feeling stress. It is considered negative and destructive. This is the stress many are experiencing with the COVID-19 pandemic. Fear of being infected, overwhelmed with negative news, changes in daily routine, or additional work or home responsibilities are creating feelings of distress.

Duration of Stress

Situational/Acute Stress. Short term stressor

Chronic Stress. Long term stressor

Note: COVID-19, like many other stressors, is a short-term, acute stress. Even though it may feel like it will last forever, it will eventually end.

EXERCISE:
Goals for Reducing Stress

Think about what your goals are for reducing stress. You can choose from the list below or add your own. Take a moment to visualize what your life will be like without this stressor in your life.

- **Medical**. Decrease the anxiety of medical procedures
- **Substance Abuse**. Issues with drugs, tobacco, and eating
- **Psychological Distress**. Control depression and anxiety
- **Physical Distress**. Reduce pain and discomfort
- **Sleep**. Reduce insomnia and enhance sleep
- **Interpersonal Stress**. Decrease interpersonal conflict
- **General Health**. Enhance general physical well-being
- **Creativity**. Enhance creativity and artistic work
- **Spirituality**. Develop spiritual growth and prayer
- **Physical Performance**. Enhance energy for sports and sex
- **Chronic Illness**. Manage diabetes and lung or heart disease

JOURNAL ENTRY

Give an example of a time you experienced each type of stress at any point in your life. Also write about an example of each from during the COVID-19 pandemic.

1. A eustress (positive, happy) event

2. A neustress (neutral) event

3. A distress (negative) event

4. An acute (short-term) stress event

5. A chronic (long-term) stress event

You have brains in your head and feet in your shoes, you can steer yourself in any direction you choose, You're on your own, and you know what you know. And YOU are the one who'll decide where to go.

- Dr. Seuss

Every disaster movie starts with the government ignoring the advice of a scientist.

LESSON 4
LESSON: The Body and Stress

Whether you realize it or not your body experiences physical reactions to stress. However, your physical symptoms may be different from other's symptoms. Becoming aware of how your body reacts to stress so you know when to use a stress reduction tool is an important part of the equation for reducing stress. Look at the following and circle the physical reactions you experience when stressed.

- Fast, hard, irregular heartbeat
- Perspiring or feeling too warm
- Hurried, shallow, or uneven breathing
- Feeling the need to use the restroom
- Tight, tense, or clenched muscles
- Feeling uncoordinated
- Restlessness and fidgetiness
- Dry mouth
- Tension and self-consciousness
- Fatigue
- Headache
- Feeling unfit or heavy
- Backache
- Shoulders, neck, or back feels tense
- Worsened skin condition
- Watering or tearing of the eyes
- Nervous or upset stomach
- Loss or increase of appetite

EXERCISE:
One Minute Body Scan

Your physical reactions to stress could be very minor. Take notice of the following stress indicators now and as you go through your day. By taking notice and using a stress tool to reduce them, you can be preventing further stress related problems.

- Am I furrowing my eyebrows?
- Am I curling my toes?
- Am I feeling tension in my arms?
- Am I clenching my jaw?
- Am I clinching my hands?
- Am I pursing my lips?
- Am I feeling tightness in my legs?
- Am I feeling tightness in my neck?
- Am I feeling shortness of breath?
- Am I hunching my shoulders?
- Do I notice tightness anywhere else?

JOURNAL ENTRY

Describe in detail how you physically react when feeling stressed. Tired? Sore? Tense? Low energy?

Describe in detail how you feel emotionally when you are stressed. Agitated? Worried? Depressed?

Describe how you feel physically and emotionally when you are at peace or happy. Calm? Joyous? Increased energy?

Experience is the hardest kind of teacher. It gives you the test first, and the lesson afterward.

- Anonymous

This is like reading a 4th grader's paper. There was a virus that attacked the world, everyone one was scared. No one left their homes or they could be arrested. The planet ran out of toilet paper, all the schools were closed, and it snowed in May.

LESSON 5
LESSON: Stress Predictors

The amount of stress created by a difficult event is determined by a number of factors, and your reaction will vary depending on your ability to handle stress.

The Covid-19 pandemic has all of the following for most people.

Unpredictability. Was the stressful event unexpected? Examples: An accident, unexpected illness, bankruptcy

Uncontrollability. Was it something over which you had little control? Examples: Weather, earthquakes, volcanic eruption

Undesirability. Was it an event that you did not want? Examples: Death of loved one, job loss, a crime

Magnitude. Was the event important or large? Examples: War, worldwide pandemic

Clustering. Did several stressful events happen at about the same time? Examples: Illness accompanied by a loss of job and divorce

EXERCISE:
Autogenic Training

Though this sounds like something superheroes would do in the movies, autogenic training is actually a relaxation therapy. It gives you the power to control various bodily functions that are normally automatic, such as heart rate, so you can override the stress response.

With autogenic training, a form of self-hypnosis developed by German neurologist Dr. J.H. Sultz, the emphasis is to make specific body parts warm and heavy, like being in a mental spa. This action relaxes the muscles by increasing blood flow from the body core to the extremities.

NOTE: You are not asleep. You are not unconscious. You will not lose control. No one controls you.

1. Take a few slow even breaths.

2. Focus attention on your arms. Quietly and slowly repeat to yourself six times, "My arms are very heavy." Then quietly say to yourself, "I am completely calm."

3. Refocus attention on your arms. Quietly and slowly repeat to yourself six times, "My arms are very warm." Then quietly say to yourself, "I am completely calm."

4. Repeat the above steps for other parts of your body. Go to your legs, head, heart, lungs, stomach, etc.

5. Enjoy the feeling of relaxation, warmth, and heaviness. When you are ready to stop, quietly say to yourself, "Arms firm, breathe deeply, eyes open."

JOURNAL ENTRY

Describe an event that caused stress in your life that was:

1. Unpredictable

2. Uncontrollable

3. Undesirable

4. Had great impact on your life

5. Had other stressors at the same time

*The journey of a thousand miles
begins with a single step.*

– Chinese proverb

Dad always said I wouldn't amount to anything lying on the sofa,
but here I am saving the world!

LESSON 6
LESSON: The "Fight, Flight, or Freeze" Response

Do you feel like you want to run out of the house screaming during the COVID-19 quarantine? Many people do. You make a choice to stay and face confrontation (fight), to run away from it (flight), and sometimes you struggle to do anything and feel stuck (freeze). But how do you fight something you cannot see, or flight from something when you cannot leave? This is accomplished by learning coping skills and stress management tools. Understand that your body is built to react to danger. It is a primitive and innate survival tactic.

Physical response to stress occurs because the sympathetic nervous system (SNS) produces changes in your body. When a stressful or dangerous situation arises, the SNS releases over thirty hormones that provides quick energy for an emergency response, such as when there is a need to run from a wild animal or an attacker.

However, everyday hassles, annoyances, and worries can also trigger fight, flight, and freeze responses. Often you are only fighting your own thoughts, but it creates the same physiological and psychological effects as real danger, and the stress hormones can build up if there is no physical release. This contributes to wear and tear on your body and can cause physical and psychological disease. But you have the ability to control this with your mind and brain.

EXERCISE: Diaphragmatic Breathing

You have heard the saying, "Just take a deep breath."

The most natural and easiest way to relax is by taking deep breaths with your diaphragm muscle, the muscle slightly above your stomach. Due to improper breathing and stress, people often use their chest to breath instead of their diaphragm which can cause increased feelings of emotion.

During diaphragmatic breathing the lower abdomen moves up and down, just like when a baby breathes.

Do the following breathing exercise.

Place your hand over your belly and the other over your chest. Do you feel your daiphragm or your chest filling with air? Keep practicing until filling your diaphragm with air comes naturally.

Inspiration and Expiration

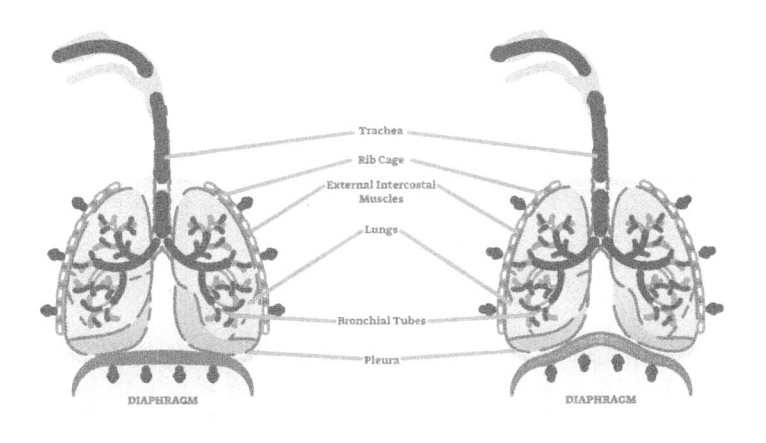

Inspiration   Expiration

JOURNAL ENTRY

Describe a time in your life when you felt like running away or fighting, or maybe you froze. How did your body react? How did your mind react?

What are the stressors you are facing today, including your thoughts about how the COVID-19 pandemic is physically and mentally affecting you? What do you feel like running from or what do you feel like fighting?

You've got to think about big things while you are doing small things, so that the small things all go in the right direction.

- Albin Toffer

To those who are complaining about the quarantine period and curfews, just remember that your grandparents were called to war, you are being called to sit on the couch and watch Netflix. You can do this.

LESSON 7
LESSON: Health and Stress

Stress can cause you to feel immediately sick or cause long-term illness. Stress can increase vulnerability to, aggravate, and prolong a wide range of illnesses including:

AIDS/HIV infection	Cancer	Heart palpitations
Pneumonia	Allergies	Chronic lung disease
Hypertension	Skin disorders	Arthritis
Cirrhosis of the liver	Influenza	Sleep disorders
Atherosclerosis	Diabetes	Irritable bowel
Stroke	Bruxism	Headache
Kidney impairment	Ulcers	

General Adaptation Syndrome (GAS) How Stress Causes Disease

Stage 1: Alarm reaction (Fight, flight, or freeze response). Body systems are activated

Stage 2: Stage of Resistance. Body tries to reach homeostasis, or normal state, but cannot

Stage 3: Stage of Exhaustion. Body parts begin to malfunction, causing disease

EXERCISE:
Hand on Belly Breathing

Extreme athletes, martial artists, and mountaineers know the importance of breathing. It is what allows them to succeed in their endeavors. Breathing is one of the quickest and most effective ways of reducing your stress.

The following exercise will teach you an additional step after diaphragmatic breathing to help you begin reducing your stress.

1. Sit or lie down and place one hand on your belly and the other on your chest.

2. Inhale through your nose making sure that the hand on your belly rises, and the hand on your chest hardly moves.

3. As you inhale slowly through your nostrils, silently count to three.

4. As you exhale through your lips, slowly count to four, feeling the hand on your belly falling gently.

5. Repeat for 5 minutes.

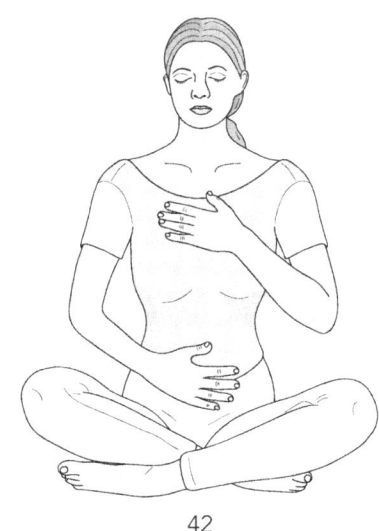

JOURNAL ENTRY

Spend a few minutes doing the deep breathing exercise. Can you feel your body relaxing?

What changes do you feel in your breathing and heart rate?

Did your emotions change after doing the breathing exercise?

How does it affect your energy level?

Choose your thoughts carefully. Keep what brings you peace and let go of what doesn't. Happiness is only one thought away.

– Nishan Panwar

Child: Dad, the lunch lady was really angry today.
Dad: Mom is under lots of stress these days.

LESSON 8
LESSON: The Mind and Stress

Your thoughts, ideas, and perceptions influence your brain and cause a physical response. You need to guard your thoughts, especially in difficult times. Unfortunately, we often think far too many negative or irrational thoughts that cause physical and psychological discomfort and disease. These thoughts lead to psychological disorders such as anxiety and depression and leave people feeling sad, angry, hopeless and helpless, lacking energy and appetite, or other symptoms.

The media coverage of the COVID-19 pandemic is full of stress producing negative information that, at times, is incorrect. Your natural response is to seek out more information to find a sense of safety. It is important that you get your information from a reliable source, such as the Center for Disease Control website. Learn to be informed but stay away from information overload.

YOU CHOOSE:

Spend your life with positive health-producing thoughts

OR

Spend your life with negative sick-producing thoughts.

EXERCISE: Alternate Nostril Breathing

This is a breathing exercise that helps you become more focused and aware of your breathing. The more aware and control you are of your breathing the more control you have of your body and mind's reaction to stress.

1. Close your eyes and focus all your attention on your breathing.

2. Begin breathing through your *right* nostril by using your finger to hold your left nostril shut. Count to three.

3. Breathe out of your *left* nostril by using your finger to hold your right nostril shut. Count to three.

4. Repeat this cycle for 20 breaths.

JOURNAL ENTRY

How do you feel when you listen to or read about news events?

What parts of it make you feel angry, depressed, or anxious? How do you feel when listening to politics? Sports? Human-interest stories?

How do you feel when you listen to news about the COVID-19 pandemic?

The best and most beautiful things in the world cannot be seen or even touched. They must be felt with the heart.

- Helen Keller

Finally getting good gas mileage – 3 weeks to the gallon.

LESSON 9
LESSON: Emotions and Stress

Emotions are defined as strong feelings. They are experienced by every culture. A fundamental difference between feelings and emotions is that feelings are experienced consciously, while emotions manifest either consciously or subconsciously. Some people may spend years, or even a lifetime, not understanding the depths of their emotions.

There are various theories on the types and number of emotions. Below is the basic list of them.

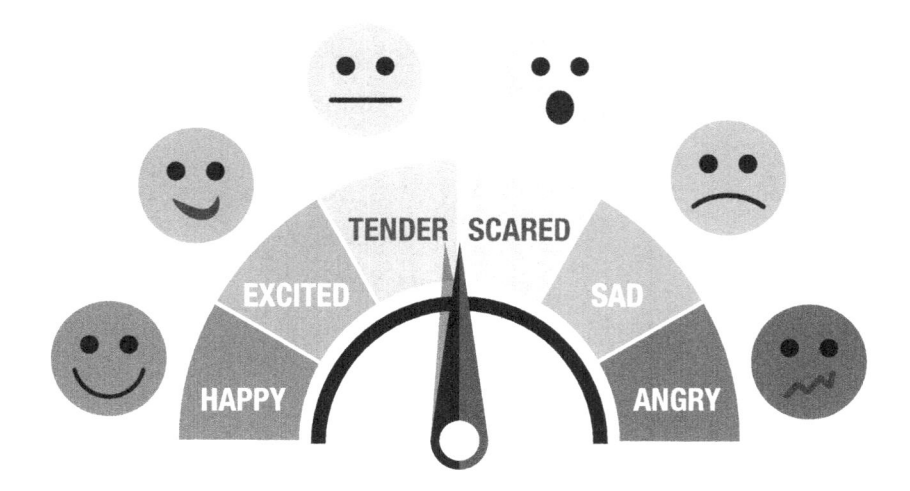

EXERCISE:
Know Your Emotions

Look at the list of emotions listed below. Practice expressing each emotion in front of a mirror. How does your face change? How does your body respond? Can you feel the emotion?

- Admiration
- Adoration
- Aesthetic Appreciation
- Amusement
- Anxiety
- Awe
- Awkwardness
- Boredom
- Calm
- Confusion
- Craving
- Disgust
- Empathetic pain
- Entranced
- Envy
- Excitement
- Fear
- Horror
- Interest
- Joy
- Nostalgia
- Romance
- Sadness
- Satisfaction
- Sexual desire
- Sympathy
- Triumph

JOURNAL ENTRY

From the list of emotions in the exercise, list any of them you have experienced today and why.

What are the emotions you are experiencing due to the COVID-19 pandemic and why?

I have had many troubles in life but the worst of them never came.

- James A. Garfield

The introverts have overtaken the world
and we must now live by their rules.

LESSON 10
LESSON: Signs that Your Mind is Stressed

Just as your body reacts to stress, your mind does too. You may feel anxious, depressed, or have difficulty concentrating when you are stressed. You may find that you have difficulty with certain mental tasks, such as problem solving or being creative.

Do you find yourself experiencing any of the following when you are stressed? Is the COVID-19 pandemic affecting you in any of the following ways?

1. Your mind seems to be racing.

2. Difficulty controlling your thoughts.

3. You are worried, irritable, sad, anxious, angry, annoyed, fearful, or upset.

4. You seem preoccupied and find concentrating more difficult.

5. You find it difficult to fall asleep, or to fall back asleep if awakened.

6. You have problems concentrating and make errors in performance.

7. You've developed a lack of creativity.

EXERCISE: Complete Breathing (Zen Breathing)

The final breathing exercise. Complete breathing is an exercise to help you gain more control and awareness of your breathing. You can also use visualization to make it more calming, such as imagining you are smelling your favorite scented flower, or blowing onto a dandelion or candle.

1. Lie Down; put one hand on your belly and the other on your chest.

2. Inhale through your nose (think of a flower that you are gently smelling) making sure that your hands rise on both your belly and chest.

3. Continue slowly inhaling through your nose first filling your belly, then lower part of your lungs, the middle part of your chest, and finally the upper part of your chest.

4. Breathe slow, even, and deep.

5. Exhale slowly through parted lips (as if gently blowing out a candle), emptying your lungs from top to bottom.

COVID-19 MENTAL SURVIVAL GUIDE

JOURNAL ENTRY

List some normal stressors you had today. What caused the stress, and what is a solution for it, so you don't have to feel this stress in the future. Do the same for stressors unique to the COVID-19 pandemic.

Normal Stressors	**What caused the stress**	**Solution**
Name a stressor	The cause	How to stop the stress

EXAMPLES

Normal Stressors	**What caused the stress**	**Solution**
Missed meeting	Time Pressure	Leave earlier
Lost wallet	Disorganized	Always leave on dresser

COVID-19 Stressors	**What caused the stress**	**Solution**
Feeling lonely	Socially isolated	Zoom meeting
Visit to public place	Needed food or supplies	Order on-line
Feeling confined	Being quarantined	Take a drive
No exercise	Gyms and parks closed	Social distance walking

Obstacles cannot crush me. Every obstacle yields to stern resolve.

- Leonardo da Vinci

Yeah, I have plans tonight.
I'll probably hit the living room around 8 or 9.

LESSON 11
LESSON: Perceptions and Attitudes

The amount of stress you experience in any given situation is largely determined by your perceptions and attitudes concerning the event. It's not about what is happening, but how you are thinking about what is happening. This is a positive thing if you maintain positive thoughts.

Your life experiences impact the way you think about events. Therefore, your perceptions and attitudes about any given situation will be different from other's perceptions and attitudes about the same situation. When you realize this, it gives you the ability to change your thoughts about events in your life.

Be an Optimist (positive) not a Pessimist (negative).

Optimism will: improve your mood; decrease depression, anxiety, and hostility; reduce physical and psychological pain; enhance the immune system and speed recovery; extend and enhance your life.

You can also be optimistic by being thankful for something in your life. If you can't find anything to be optimistic about, you probably aren't looking hard enough.

EXERCISE:
Guided Imagery

Guided imagery is using words or music to create a desired state of being with a beneficial effect. It has health-related benefits that can be physical and emotional. With guided imagery a person can lower their stress levels; help achieve an athletic, academic, or career goal; promote healing; manage pain; or quit an addictive behavior.

Listen to a guided imagery on the internet or your favorite app. Or close your eyes to create your own 5-10 minute images and journey within your mind. Create a daydream or fantasy of a relaxing situation.

Put no effort into directing where thought goes. Simply allow it to go where it would like to go.

Remain passive. Do nothing but note the relaxing sensations.

Use this to prepare for the day or unwind from the day.

JOURNAL ENTRY

Make a list of places you would like to go in your mind. Maybe it is somewhere you have been, a favorite spot as a child, a place you would like to visit, another planet, or somewhere else in your imagination.

From one choice on your list, write a short guided imagery script. Describe the sights, sounds, smells, and anything else you want to experience, and what you see yourself doing.

Happiness, wealth, and success are the by-products of goal setting. They cannot be the goal themselves.

- Denis Waitley

What do you call panic-buying of sausage and cheese in Germany? The wurst-kase scenario.

LESSON 12
LESSON: Values and Goals

Values are the principles and qualities that are important to you. You have values for Family and Home, Financial and Career, Spiritual and Ethical, Physical and Health, Social and Cultural, Mental and Educational.

For a comprehensive list of values, see the List Of Values at the end of the book.

Has the COVID-19 pandemic changed your values? Is family time more important than before? Do you find yourself being more appreciative and thankful?

Goals are real and specific. They are what you are aiming to achieve with your time, resources, and life.

Your goals may have changed since the start of the pandemic. Make sure the goal you are working for is something you really want and value.

EXERCISE:
Guided Imagery II

Close your eyes and take yourself on a 15 minute Guided Imagery journey. You can imagine lying under the stars, looking at clouds, going on a hike, a childhood experience, or anything else that would bring you relaxation. Don't forget to follow the guided imagery rules from the previous lesson.

JOURNAL ENTRY

Choose your values from the list in the back of this book.

Now write your personal and professional goals. Next to them write the values they each express.

Never put off until tomorrow what you can do today.

- Thomas Jefferson

I don't think anyone expected that when we changed the clocks we'd go from Standard Time to Twilight Zone

LESSON 13
LESSON: Time and Stress

Depending on your situation, whether you are the CEO of a major corporation, a health care worker, stay at home with your children, or unemployed, time management is important. If you're a really busy person, time management can help you get organized, prioritize, and decrease your stress. If you find yourself in a transitional phase with not much to do, time management will help you focus and be more productive, which in turn will reduce your stress.

Here are several tips for being more effective with your time management. When doing your tasks:

1. Do the most difficult or unpleasant first.

2. Finish one task and then start the other task.

3. Break big jobs into smaller jobs.

4. If you must wait to finish a job, resume it as quickly as possible. Humans are poor multi-taskers.

5. Overestimate your time to complete a task.

6. Don't waste time planning – START DOING IT!

7. Avoid unproductive work.

8. Complete all tasks.

9. Continue monitoring the use of your time.

NOTE – See the Time Management worksheet in the LOGS section in the back of the book to help organize your time and tasks.

EXERCISE:
Urgent/Important Principle

To effectively manage your time you must know which tasks are important and which ones are urgent. The Eisenhower Urgent/Important Principle helps you organize which tasks need to be done and when.

The worksheet for this exercise is included in the back of the book.

Important activities have an outcome that leads to achieving your personal and professional goals.

Urgent activities demand immediate attention, are usually being demanded by another individual, and have consequences if they are not completed.

List all the things you need to do and prioritize them according to their importance and urgency.

1. **Urgent and Important.** Important tasks that must be done now. Example: crises, application for school or job, etc.

2. **NOT Urgent but Important.** Important tasks, but you can wait to do them. Example: regular maintenance, creating a budget, buying groceries.

3. **Urgent but NOT Important.** Tasks that aren't important but need to be done. Example: regular meetings and phone calls.

4. **NOT Urgent and NOT Important.** Tasks that aren't important and don't need to be done. Example: social media, unimportant phone calls, time wasting activities.

JOURNAL ENTRY

Describe where you feel you are pressed for time. How does your body feel when you are pressed for time?

What thoughts do you have when you don't have enough time?

What are you going to do to better manage your time?

*It is not enough to be busy, so are the ants.
The question is: What are we busy about?*

- Henry David Thoreau

What types of jokes are allowed during quarantine? Inside jokes!

LESSON 14
LESSON: Pareto Principle (80/20 Rule)

The Pareto Principle, also known as the 80/20 rule, named after economist Vilfredo Pareto, specifies that on average 20% of your work results in 80% of your results. This implies that you could be much more productive with 80% of your time.

You can use this principle to identify which 20% of your customers are bringing in 80% of your sales. Or what 20% in your life is causing 80% of your distractions.

The goal is to spend more of your time being productive so you can achieve greater results, thus having more time and less stress in your life.

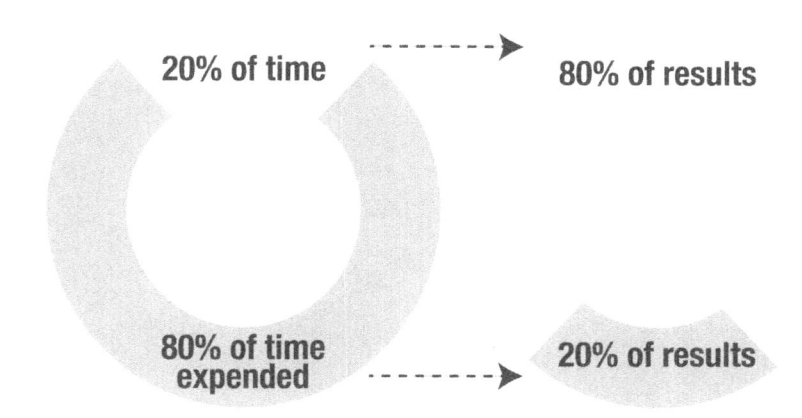

20% of time ┈┈┈▶ **80% of results**

80% of time expended ┈┈┈▶ **20% of results**

EXERCISE:
Using the Pareto Principle

The purpose of the Pareto Principle for time management is to prioritize your to-do list in order of time and effort versus the rewards you receive.

Start by making a list of tasks by order of effort and rewards. Now order them by those requiring the least effort with the greatest results.

Those that deliver the greatest results with the least effort are completed first. Others that require more effort with little results can be postponed or removed from your to-do list.

For example: If you had a list of 10 tasks, the first 2 on the list will probably give you 80% of your results with only 20% of your effort or time. The other 8 items will require 80% of your time and give you only 20% of your results.

JOURNAL ENTRY

If you could, how would you spend your perfect day where you felt productive 100% of the time?

What work would you do?

How would you spend your leisure time?

Who would you enjoy working and living around?

The secret to getting ahead is getting started.

- Mark Twain

I need to practice social distancing from the refrigerator.

LESSON 15
LESSON: Procrastination

Not all people who procrastinate are procrastinators. True procrastinators put things off to the detriment of their own well-being.

Procrastination is waiting to start tasks that needs to be done by a particular time when there's no good reason for the delay. You typically have a small window of time before you must begin the task, but at some point your avoidance raises your stress levels and causes physiological and psychological distress. This results in undesirable effects such as sleeplessness and anxiety.

The sooner you take action, the less anxiety you will feel, and you will find an improvement in your emotional and physical well-being.

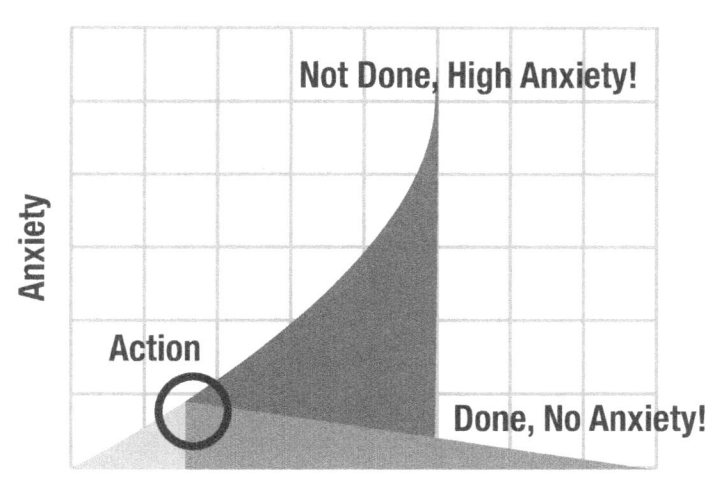

EXERCISE:
Stop Procrastinating

Here are steps to help you stop procrastinating and eliminating stress caused by deadlines.

1. Get organized. Get a planner.

2. Divide tasks into simple steps. Baby steps make it easier.

3. Schedule time to do the task.

4. Set a specific deadline. "Someday" is not a deadline.

5. Get rid of any distractions. Put away your phone.

6. Keep track of your time and productivity.

7. Take a break. Your mind and body need and deserve it.

8. Incentivize yourself. Choose incentives that are positive, healthy, and inspirational.

9. Do the hard tasks first. Other tasks will look easier.

10. Let people know your goals for completion. Be accountable.

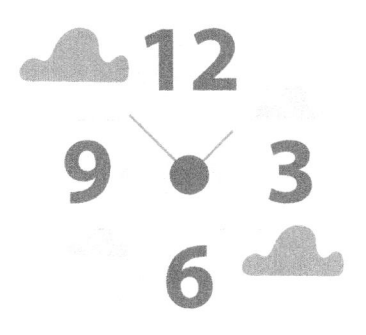

JOURNAL ENTRY

What is a project you have been procrastinating? How do you feel while putting it off?

Go do the project. How did you feel when you were doing it? How do you feel now that you have completed the project?

What are some tips you can write down to help yourself not procrastinate the next time you have a project? Ideas include reminding yourself how good it feels to get things done.

People are as happy as they make up their minds to be.

- Abraham Lincoln

Never in my wildest of wild dreams did I ever think I would go up to a bank teller and request money with a mask on.

LESSON 16
LESSON: Financial Stress

Financial concerns are one of the leading causes of stress. In a world where financial certainty is rarely guaranteed, people worry and stress about how they will pay their bills, have food to eat or a place to live, pay for their child's education, and cover necessary medical expenses.

Financial stress is linked to health problems like anxiety, depression, marital problems, sleep disorders, excessive worrying, drinking, smoking and overeating.

The COVID-19 pandemic has created financial stress for people around the world. Even prior to the pandemic, research stated that over half of all workers had money problems. The pandemic has exacerbated this problem, also causing an increase in mental and physical health problems.

Signs of financial problems

Little or no savings	Making minimum payments
Always use credit	Unclear of debt owed
At or near credit limit	Bounced checks
Take cash advances	Collectors calling
Denied credit	

EXERCISE: Create a Budget

It is easy to create a quick budget so you know where your money is coming from and where it is going. Don't let fear or worry get in the way of creating your budget. You will have less stress when you know your financial situation instead of living in denial about it. You may even find you are in a much better situation than you thought. Either way, having a budget will give you more control over your money and help decrease your financial stress.

Steps to creating a quick and easy budget:

1. List all your sources of income and their amounts.

2. List all your expenses, including mortgage or rental payments, utility bills, automobile expenses, food, app subscriptions, everything!

3. Take the total from #1 and subtract the total of #2. This amount is what you have left over.

4. Decide what you really *need* and what you just *want*.

5. Add all your needs together to try to reduce #2.

6. Subtract your needs from your income. Try to have more income than expenses. This is your budget.

7. Stick to your budget and make adjustments as necessary.

8. Put extra money into needs, savings, and investments.

9. Plan for future items and expenses using the 50/30/20 method. This method suggests allocating your money to 50% needs / 30% wants / 20% savings.

JOURNAL ENTRY

List your revenue and expenses. What are your financial concerns (positive and negative) and how do each of them make you feel and cause a disruption to your life?

Create a financial plan by getting information about how you can make payment arrangements, get loans or assistance, or consider what you can do without at this time. Also, is there something you can do to increase your income?

After doing this exercise write about how doing it changed your stress levels regarding your finances, and what adjustments you can continue to make to reduce stress.

It's not stress that kills us, it is our reaction to it.

- Hans Selye, Stress Researcher

Want to find the cure for Coronavirus fast?
Keep the schools closed. The parents will be on it!

LESSON 17
LESSON: Organizational Stress

Mess means stress! Your home should provide you a sanctuary from stress. A cluttered or disorganized living space or office will cause additional stress. In fact, just sitting in a cluttered room can cause stress reactions in your system.

On the other hand, being in a space characterized by order, tranquility, and your unique tastes can soothe and relax you. You will feel more empowered by your environment when you aren't constantly losing important papers, walking amongst a clutter of unpacked boxes and piles on your desk, and unsure of finances. Take control of your space! Get rid of stuff you don't need and set aside time to organize your life. You will feel more in control and less stressed.

Now is the perfect time to start! If you are staying home because of the COVID-19 pandemic, you now have time to get your home or business more organized.

EXERCISE: Steps to Getting Organized

Do the following to help you get organized:

1. Decide what you need to organize. Is it your time, office, or home?

2. Do not procrastinate or let things stop you.

3. Organize your time in a planner or calendar.

4. Do one chore at a time.

5. De-clutter one space at a time.

6. Get others to help if you need it, for example professional cleaners.

7. Get rid of things you don't need and stop doing things that waste your time.

8. Don't bring in more stuff or add more things that will just end up being a distraction.

9. Label boxes, create files, organize computer files, etc.

10. Put things away when you use them.

11. Check off items you have accomplished.

12. Create a system so you are no longer unorganized and overwhelmed.

13. Enjoy your organized stress-free life!

JOURNAL ENTRY

List areas of your life that are cluttered or disorganized. What problems does disorganization cause you? What are you going to do to get organized?

Disorganized area

Problems caused by being disorganized

When and how to organize it

We live longer than our forefathers, but we suffer more from a thousand artificial anxieties and cares. They fatigued only the muscles; we exhaust the finer strength of the nerves.

- Edward George

Me: This show is boring.
My Boss: This is a Zoom conference.

LESSON 18
LESSON: Work Stress

Work is a leading cause of stress. Deadlines, Long hours, heavy workloads, job insecurity, and feeling a lack of purpose creates stress.

Many are experiencing job stress during the COVID-19 pandemic. Healthcare workers, truck drivers, businesses, and many others are either having to work harder and longer hours or having to restructure their business to accommodate new regulations.

Ideas that will help you manage and cope with job stress:

1. Identify your symptoms of work stress. Anxiety? Overwhelmed?

2. Identify the sources of your work stress. Be objective. No finger-pointing.

3. Identify how you respond to your work stressors. Be an observer of yourself.

4. Set goals to respond more effectively to your work stress.

5. Motivate yourself with inspiring music, videos, apps, exercise, or a positive book.

6. Change your thinking. See how others are solving similar problems.

7. Talk with your supervisor regarding your direction in the company, your strengths, and their expectations for you.

8. When in conflict, negotiate. Have someone mediate for you.

9. Pace and balance yourself.

10. Know when to quit and move on to the next item. Come back to it later.

EXERCISE: Making SMART Goals

Recall your goals from the meditations you did in previous lessons. Write them down using the SMART method for goal achievement.

Specific. Clearly define your goal. Answer the questions who, what, when, why, and where.

Measurable. Set progress markers within your goal.

Achievable. Be ambitious, but not outrageous.

Relevant. Make sure your goal is in line with your long-term vision for yourself or your company

Timebound. Use specific deadlines

Examples

I will find one new hobby, read one book, or learn one new skill by next week.

I will practice meditation every morning for five minutes.

I will lose five pounds in four weeks by exercising at the gym two times per week.

JOURNAL ENTRY

What is the source of your work stress?

How does it make you feel?

How do you physically and mentally react to work stress?

How can you minimize or eliminate some of your stress in your work environment and in your thinking?

There are times when we stop, we sit still. We listen, and breezes from a whole other world begin to whisper.

- James Carroll

My children's homeschool courses: AP Chores, Honor Yard Work, Dishwashing 101, Physical Education Trash Removal, and extra credit for Laundry.

LESSON 19
LESSON: Working from Home

Working from home can be easy for some and difficult and stressful for others.

If you or are suddenly forced to work from home because you lost your job, got injured, or as has happened to many recently because of the COVID-19 pandemic, your routine can be shattered.

Maybe you don't have the readily available resources you had at your office. It's possible your social support and business networks are disrupted or even non-existent. You may have distractions, such as children who are on break from school. For many reasons, working from home can be completely different from working in an office.

Though you may find there are things you don't have control over, there are some you do. An incredibly beneficial tool you can use is establishing a work-from-home routine. Studies show that having established routines increases productivity and reduces stress and stress-related problems.

EXERCISE: Work/Time Routine

It's time to go to work! You must continue using the skills that make you productive at the office while you are at home. Doing the following will help you maintain a routine, increase your productivity and reduce your stress levels.

1. Clean-up and get dressed. Don't dress sloppy. Groom yourself like you would if you were going to the office. Brush your hair and teeth. And please, put some pants on during the video call.

2. Create a designated space to focus and work. Personalize it with pictures, good lighting, a comfortable chair, necessary technology, and places to store and organize office necessities.

3. Avoid distractions. Don't watch the news, videos, or run the errands. Protect your work day for work.

4. Socialize. Spend time video chatting with business associates. Seeing a face is better than texting.

5. Stick to your routine. You have a work-day routine at the office, do the same at home. However, allow yourself to sneak a kiss to your spouse and hug your kids while joining them for lunch or a quick playtime. These are definite benefits to working at home. Take advantage of it and feel the rewards!

JOURNAL ENTRY

Starting with the beginning of your work day, list every activity you need to do, including getting ready for work, necessary tasks and phone calls you need to make, and completing your work day.

What do you need to do to have the perfect office space at home? What technology should you purchase? Do you need pictures for your walls or desk?

Anyone can become angry, that is easy. But to be angry with the right person, to the right degree, at the right time, for the right purpose, and in the right way ---this is not easy.

- Aristotle

Why does leaving the house feel like I am making a supply run on the show Walking Dead?

LESSON 20
LESSON: Anger and Stress

Everyone feels anger. It is a normal emotion. Though feeling anger is normal, how you handle it makes a great difference in the outcomes of situations. Your response to your own emotions can either make the situation or relationship worse, or help toward healing it.

The COVID-19 pandemic has many people who are normally happy and easy-going feeling short-tempered and irritated. Anger is a reaction to a perceived pain, frustration, or worry that is often projected toward others. It is also an expression of stress. This can be detrimental to your health. Research shows anger causes heart attacks and strokes and weakens your immune system.

Many people know they need to handle their anger better and learning to calm yourself when you start to feel angry is a great way to do this. Try to recognize your "triggers" for anger. Triggers are situations or events that cause you to feel a particular way. When you know your triggers you can be better prepared to remain calm when these situations arise. By properly managing anger you will find you can reduce or eliminate it.

Meditation

Meditation is a practice by which individuals use specific techniques to focus their mind and thoughts. People use it to increase their awareness of themselves and their surroundings. Meditation is used to reduce stress and symptoms of anger. It also creates emotional calm and promotes mental clarity. There are several meditation techniques including mindfulness, yoga, loving-kindness, and guided meditation.

EXERCISE:
Practice Meditation

Calmly attend to a simple stimulus (a word like *one* or your breathing) without thought, analysis, or effort.

Calmly return your attention to your thought after every distraction.

Continue to gently return your focus from distractions for 10 minutes.

If you want to practice a Loving Meditation add good thoughts toward yourself and others, especially those you feel have hurt you. You can say phrases like, "May I be happy. May I be peaceful and at ease. May you be well. May you be safe."

JOURNAL ENTRY

Write about something or somebody who made you angry. What was happening, and do these situations tend to cause you to feel anger whenever they happen? These are your "triggers."

What were your emotions before, during, and after you experienced anger?

How could you have handled the situation differently?

Do a loving meditation about someone who angers you. Describe the experience you had during and after the meditation.

Listening is an art that requires attention over talent, spirit over ego, others over self.

- Dean Jackson

Day 3 without sports. Found a lady sitting on my couch yesterday. Apparently she is my wife. She seems nice.

LESSON 21
LESSON: Couple's Stress

Even in the best of times, romantic relationships have their challenges. A healthy, supportive relationship takes work. It can be difficult, but it is well worth the time, patience, and love you put into it.

Couples are finding the COVID-19 pandemic has caused new relationship challenges to surface. They have had to make adjustments to being quarantined apart, or constantly together; compromise on their differing opinions of what social distancing should look like; divide new household responsibilities so nobody feels overwhelmed or unfairly treated.

When you find yourself in the midst of conflict, improved communication can be the key to working it out, and being a good listener is the most important part of good communication. Different listening styles include:

Competitive or combative listening: People want to push their own opinion rather than listen to their partner. This is a good way to start an argument.

Passive, attentive listening: People are interested, but not really understanding what their partner is saying.

Active, reflective listening: People actively listen and understand what the other person is saying.

EXERCISE: Active Listening

Active listening involves concentrating on what is being said by the speaker rather than just passively 'hearing' their message. To do this you must listen with all your senses.

1. Give the speaker your full attention. Look at them directly and focus on what they are saying. Make sure you aren't just mentally preparing a rebuttal while they are speaking. Watch their body language. Non-verbal language can be louder than words.

2. Let them know you are listening. Have a posture that is open and interested. Nod and give verbal cues you hear them, such as saying, "yes."

3. Provide Feedback. Occasionally paraphrase or summarize their ideas by responding with, "What I just heard you say is…" You can also ask questions for clarification.

4. Do not judge, criticize, interrupt, or argue with the speaker. Listen with an open heart and mind. This is a critical component in your ability to come up with a compromise.

5. Respond Appropriately. Once you have really listened, and only then, should you reply. Reply with respect and honesty. Have the goal of working with the other person to find the most positive and loving solutions.

JOURNAL ENTRY

What type of communicator are you? Competitive, passive, or active? Give examples of when you have been each of them.

What type of communicator is your partner? How does their communication style make you feel?

What type of communicator is your employer or co-worker? How does their communication style make you feel?

Kids are like a mirror, what they see and hear they do. Be a good reflection for them.

- Kevin Heath

If there's a baby boom nine months from now, what will happen in 2033? There will be a whole bunch of quaranteens.

LESSON 22
LESSON: Parenting Stress

Children and teens will react to stress based on how those around them are reacting to it. It is important for parents to act calmly and confidently to provide the best support for their children. Like the oxygen mask on the plane, the more secure and prepared you are, the more secure your children will feel. Use the tools in this course to help you with this.

Pay attention to these symptoms if you notice them in your child since the beginning of the COVID-19 pandemic.

- Uncharacteristic behaviors, acting out
- Illicit drugs or alcohol use
- Sleeping problems or night terrors
- Feelings of depression, or extended periods of sadness
- Complaints of physical pain or headaches
- Crying more than usual
- Increase in bedwetting, or more needy than usual
- Avoidance of usual activities
- Academics are suffering

If your child is exhibiting these behaviors it is important to call your doctor. You can also seek the advice of a therapist who specializes in child behavior and family counseling. This can be extremely helpful in providing both short and long-term solutions.

EXERCISE:
Parent Communication

Communicating with your child can be challenging at times. It is important to talk with your child or teen about stressful events that can make them anxious, including issues about the COVID-19 pandemic.

Do your best to answer their questions while reassuring them that they are safe.

Focus on prevention and the importance of following the rules for social distancing during the pandemic.

Limit your family's exposure to news coverage, social media, and other sources of negative and potentially inaccurate information. Give them accurate information.

Make life as normal as possible for them.

Create a comfortable learning environment for them to study or interact with their friends online.

Find fun activities to do as a family and for them to do on their own. Try to keep up with regular routines. Don't be too busy to have family time.

Find ways they can be outside. Maybe working in the yard or helping a neighbor.

Be a role model. What you do is more important than what you say.

JOURNAL ENTRY

What do you normally discuss with your child or teen? What are some of the questions they ask? What comments do they make about you, their friends, and the world?

Is your child anxious? If so, what are they anxious about?

What has worked to reduce your child's anxiety in the past? Can you repeat any of these actions now?

Every good thought you think is contributing its share to the ultimate result of your life.

- Grenville Kleiser

Stay optimistic.
Rapunzel met her husband while being quarantined.

LESSON 23
LESSON: Relationship Stress

Humans are social creatures and must have healthy social relationships. Having a spouse, good friends, or a loving pet can decrease your stress, increase your immune system and physical and mental health, and prolong your life. However, toxic relationships can have the opposite effect and be destructive to your physical, mental, and social health.

The COVID-19 pandemic is causing relationship problems with significant others, supervisors, children, friends, and co-workers. The following suggestions will help you cope more skillfully with the stresses in relationships:

1. Practice active listening. Develop your ability to listen more empathetically using techniques in the Active Listening exercise in this book.

2. Focus on defeating the problem(s) not the person.

3. See conflict as having the potential for being useful. It can stimulate discussion and promote positive changes in relationships. Conflict can bring people closer.

4. Create an environment in which all parties feel able to be open and honest about feelings, opinions, and facts. Work together to solve problems and create solutions.

5. Look for solutions that are acceptable to everyone.

EXERCISE:
Quick Calming Techniques

When people get angry they need to immediately calm themselves so they can think and behave in a more positive, productive way. Practice the following to quickly calm yourself. Find the ones that work best for you.

1. Take 10 deep diaphragmatic breaths through your nose.

2. Think of being somewhere else like a beach, hiking, or with loved ones.

3. Picture the other person doing something funny, like dressing strangely, brushing their teeth in an odd way, or making a goofy face.

4. Think and act from a place of being the most loving person you can be. Think to yourself, "What are the most loving words or actions I can use at this moment."

5. Agree to walk away and come back in 45 minutes – the amount of time it takes for cooler heads to prevail.

6. Do all the above together.

IMPORTANT: Remember, it is *your* thinking, not theirs, that determines how you react.

JOURNAL ENTRY

Think about the people in your life, past and present, who have emotionally helped or hurt you and look for any patterns in your relationships. Also, think about if there is anything YOU can do better.

People who have helped me

People who have hurt me

What is something positive I learned from each of these relationships?

What can I say or do to express gratitude for each of the above listed individuals? Say, "Thank you and I love you" in your mind to each of them.

Be determined to handle any challenge in a way that will make you grow.

- Les Brown

I am 30 minutes into homeschooling my 6-year-old.
I suggest that all schoolteachers are paid
one million dollars per year from now on.

LESSON 24
LESSON: Caregiver Stress – Compassion Fatigue

Being a caregiver can be stressful for anyone during normal times. Caregiver burnout is a state of physical, emotional, and mental exhaustion. Stressed caregivers may experience fatigue, anxiety, and depression. Healthcare workers, mental health professionals, and others are finding the COVID-19 pandemic extremely stressful for them professionally and personally. Parents taking care of children as well as adults taking care of elderly parents are having to work overtime and are being stressed physically and mentally.

Caregivers must be aware and take precautions to reduce feeling burnt out. It can cause physical and mental problems for the caregiver, which in turn makes it difficult to compassionately care for the ones we love.

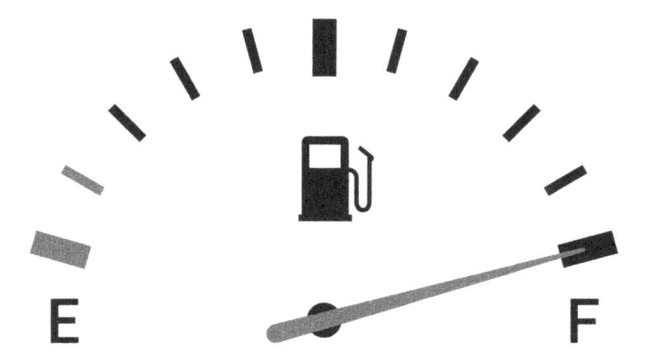

Think of it like a gas tank. If your tank is empty, how can you add fuel to another's tank? Recognize the value and importance of taking the time to fill your own tank so you have plenty to give to others. That may seem hard to do when you have so much on your plate, but you will find you feel better and more refreshed as you tackle your day, and others will feel the benefits of your improved mental state.

EXERCISE:
Avoiding Caregiver Burnout

The Cleveland Clinic offers some suggestions on how to avoid feeling overwhelmed as a caregiver.

- Talk to someone you trust about your situation and how you feel.
- Set realistic goals, accept that you may need help with care giving, and turn to others for help with some tasks.
- Take advantage of respite care services. Respite care provides a temporary break for caregivers.
- Practice self-care by setting aside time for yourself.
- Talk to a professional such as therapists, social workers, or clergy members.
- Know your limits. Don't be shy about asking for help if you can't do something.
- Develop your coping skills. Find something to be thankful about and look for the humor in life.
- Stay healthy by eating right and getting plenty of exercise and sleep.
- It's okay to feel angry or frustrated, but it's not okay to beat yourself up over it.
- Join or create a caregiver support network.

JOURNAL ENTRY

Journal how you feel when you are helping others. What have you learned about yourself and life by caring for others?

What do you find most challenging when caring for others?

What are some steps you can begin taking TODAY to fill your own fuel tank? Exercise? Eating healthier? Joining a support giver network?

You're good enough, you're smart enough, and gosh darn it people like you.

- Stuart Smalley (fictional character played by Al Franken in SNL)

People with a cold: "I just want to stay in bed and do nothing. I feel terrible."

People with coronavirus:
"I feel terrible, I think I will go skiing in Austria, visit the Eiffel Tower, and maybe do some white water rafting in Camino de Santiago."

LESSON 25
LESSON: The ABC's of Stress Management

This is a simple way to manage your stress.

A – The stressor that you are experiencing, for example a deadline, a presentation, or parenting.

B – Your *belief* about **A**, which typically shows up in a fear you have about it, such as a fear of being laughed at, a fear of losing your job, or a fear of your kids growing up and being drug addicts.

C – The amount of change you experience from thinking about the stressor, such as a racing heart or feeling panicky or irritable.

You can usually change A, B, or C.

Examples of changing A

Always late? Use time management tips from this course. Fear of presentations? Join Toastmasters. Parenting fears? Take parenting classes or read articles online.

If you can't change A then change B

Look for instances in your past to dispute your beliefs. Replace pessimistic thinking with optimistic thoughts.

If you can't change A or B, then change C

Change your thoughts and emotions by practicing relaxation techniques you're learning in this course to reduce feelings of stress.

EXERCISE: Thought Stopping

Thought Stopping is a beneficial method that quickly eliminates unwanted and stress-producing worries and concerns. When practiced, it can be a very effective way of keep out unwanted thoughts by replacing them with positive and pleasant thoughts. You can use Thought Stopping techniques whenever you have a negative thought about the COVID-19 pandemic.

There are several Thought Stopping techniques.

Classic Stop Thought Technique

- Notice your thoughts.
- Create a stop sign in your mind.
- Yell "STOP!'
- Do it every time the thought appears.
- Find a replacement thought that is relaxing and peaceful to you.

Other Stop Thought Techniques

- Snap a rubber band on your wrist.
- Replace "I can't" with "I will."
- Scattered counting. Count to 20 by scattering the numbers, 3,17,11,13,5, ...

Preoccupy your mind with something else

- Listen to a podcast, music, or an inspirational or calming app.
- Follow positive or humorous accounts on your social media, or read a good book.

COVID-19 MENTAL SURVIVAL GUIDE

JOURNAL ENTRY

Write about a stressor you've had in the past or are experiencing right now.

Use the **ABC model** to write about different ways of reducing the stress. What practical steps can you take to help you feel empowered over the stressor?

What has happened in your past that disproves your fears?

What are some relaxation techniques you can use to reduce your stress? What is a different, more positive way you can look at the situation?

TODD HUSTON

A pessimist is one who makes difficulties of his opportunities, and an optimist is one who makes opportunities of his difficulties.

- Harry Truman

Stay inside, practice social distancing, clean yourself regularly. I think I've become a house cat.

LESSON 26
LESSON:
De-Stress Engineering

Engineers are problem solvers. Prior to the COVID-19 pandemic studies reported that over 80% of Americans admitted to feeling stressed. The pandemic has caused a steep rise in these numbers. Be a de-stress engineer. With this stress tool you can find solutions to the problems that cause you to stress.

Look at all the variables that are causing, or you think are causing, your stress. This includes external and internal causes. External includes anything in your environment that causes a problem, such as deadlines, family members, or uncooperative team members. Internal includes negative characteristics within you, such as being easily angered, or a tendency to procrastinate.

Be objective. Look at yourself, others, and environmental causes, some which may seem out of your control. Then get to work at developing a solution. You will do better if you maintain a positive attitude and refrain from judging yourself and others.

Use this simple step-by-step process to solve stressful problems you face in your life and during the COVID-19 pandemic.

EXERCISE:
Solution Focused Visualization

Stress engineering is about finding solutions. Choose a problem or stressor you are experiencing and generate alternatives and solutions using stress engineering. Be creative and open to all suggestions.

1. Define your stressor. Think about a stressor you are dealing with right now.

2. Identify your initial response. Afraid, hurt, depressed, resentful, angry?

3. Generate alternatives. Think about the possible solutions to eliminate the stressor, even if that solution includes *you* needing to change.

4. Choose the best solution. Pick the solution that will work best.

5. Evaluate your choice. Did you get an acceptable outcome? If not, try again. Generate new alternatives (step 3) and try them out. Repeat this until you achieve an outcome you feel comfortable with.

JOURNAL ENTRY

Write about a problem you think the stress engineering model could solve. Besides stress, what are your emotions about it?

List some of the solutions you think would be beneficial.

How much do you want to find solutions to this stressor? Write about how your life will be different once you figure out solutions.

He who cannot change the very fabric of his thought will never be able to change reality.

- Anwar Sadat

Is this real-world Jumanji? A world-wide virus pandemic, full moon, Friday the 13th, and Daylight Savings Time all in the same week!

LESSON 27
LESSON: Survival Strategies for Life-Threatening Stressors

The Veterans Administration recommends using some of the same strategies to reduce stress during the COVID-19 pandemic that are used to survive life-threatening situations. Following are strategies recommended for life-threatening situations.

1. Quickly recognize, acknowledge, and accept the reality of the situation.

2. Make a plan for dealing with feelings of being overwhelmed or overly distressed. Preparation can make you feel more in control if these feelings arise and help you move through them quickly.

3. Combat unhelpful emotions by using distractions or staying busy – both mentally and physically.

4. Avoid impulsive behavior.

5. Get organized.

6. Increase positive coping behaviors that have worked in the past.

7. Shift negative self-statements to statements that allow you to function with less distress. Try changing "this is a terrible time" to "this is a terrible time, but I can get through this."

8. Rather than getting discouraged, focus on what you can accomplish or control.

9. Seek out mentoring or information to improve your ability to make decisions and take actions when necessary.

10. Try to engage in the situation as a challenge to be met, which can increase your ability to act both creatively and decisively.

EXERCISE:
Fear vs. Danger

Fear is what you experience in your mind because of something you believe about a situation. Danger is a real consequence of a situation, not just what you think could happen, or how you feel about what you think could happen.

When you let go of the fear and focus on the danger you are able to see the truth of the situation more clearly. Doing this allows you to make better decisions and take proper action to minimize or eliminate the danger. This creates a safer, less stressful environment for you and others.

Think of something you have recently feared, or are now fearing, such as the COVID-19 pandemic. Write it at the top of a sheet of paper. Make two columns, one labeled FEAR and the other DANGER.

1. List everything you fear about the situation under the fear column.

2. List all the dangers under the danger column.

3. List solutions to the situation based on the real dangers you listed.

JOURNAL ENTRY

Write down your fears and fears you've had in the past.

Which fears came true?

Write down one of your fears and describe the danger that creates your fear. What can you do to eliminate the danger? If you were to eliminate the danger, would you still fear it?

Ordinary people think of spending time. Great people think of using it.

- Anonymous

PSA: Every two days try your jeans on to make sure they still fit. Pajamas will have you believing all is well in the kingdom.

LESSON 28
LESSON: Physical Activity

Exercise reduces stress. The stress hormones released in your body during fight, flight, or freeze are eliminated when you fight or flee. When you freeze, or do nothing, they sit in your system and can cause unhealthy physical and mental symptoms. People have many excuses for not making time for physical activity: work, children, errands, being bored, too tired, etc.

The COVID-19 pandemic makes working out more difficult for most people. Even if you do not have exercise equipment at home, there are still exercises you can do at home and work. You want to accumulate 30 minutes or more of moderate-intensity physical activity most days of the week. Besides lowering stress and anxiety levels, moderate physical activity can:

- Reduce risk of coronary heart disease and stroke
- Increase your overall physical and mental health, including anxiety and depression
- Help with creativity and problem solving
- Raise "good" artery-clearing HDL cholesterol
- Help control blood pressure
- Decrease risk of osteoporosis and diabetes
- Help control weight and the problems associated with obesity
- Possibly protect against cancer of the colon, breast, ovaries, and cervix

EXERCISE:
Exercise to Reduce Stress

Exercise has a tranquilizing effect that reduces anxiety more effectively than many medications, or even quiet rest. People that exercise find their moods elevated. Exercise produces a longer-lasting sense of relaxation than does an equal amount of time spent practicing a relaxation technique.

You don't need a gym to stay healthy. The following are ideas for physical activities you can do without exercise equipment.

- Climbing steps
- Cycling
- Dancing
- Gardening
- General calisthenics
- House cleaning
- Painting the walls or a fence
- Playing with children
- Raking leaves
- Running
- Walking briskly
- Washing windows
- Washing the car
- Playing frisbee
- Taking the dog for a walk

Use your imagination, enjoy some activities, and reap the benefits!

JOURNAL ENTRY

List some physical activities you enjoyed as a child.

What can you do to make your physical activities more enjoyable now?

What are some physical activities you would like to do but never learned? Be creative!

Dreams...the royal road to the unconscious.

- Sigmund Freud

And you thought dogs were hard to train! It's almost impossible to get a human to "sit" and "stay."

LESSON 29
LESSON: Sleep and Stress

Stress can cause sleepless nights, which affects you and those around you. When you can't turn off your anxious thoughts and feelings it can be hard to get to sleep and stay asleep. Research shows it is important to get 7-9 hours of sleep each night for your physical and mental health.

Experts believe that almost half of all sleep problems are due to stress. Signs of sleep deprivation include: dozing off, needing an alarm clock, sleeping late, slowed thinking and reacting, difficulty understanding directions or remembering information, making mistakes, having poor attention, feeling depressed, having a negative mood, being impatient or quick to anger.

Tips for better sleeping

- Skip caffeine, alcohol, and nicotine
- Exercise before 6:00 pm
- Sleep in a dark, cool room (60-70 degrees) that is quiet
- Read or write before bedtime – avoid stimulating media
- Take a hot bath before bedtime
- Wake at the same time every day
- Only use the bedroom for sleep, relaxing, or pleasurable activities

EXERCISE:
Dream Therapy

Dreams can reveal where you have stress in your life. Try remembering your dreams by writing about them.

1. Keep a pad of paper and pen beside your bed.

2. Relax your body and review your day.

3. Repeat, "When I wake up, I will remember my dream."

4. If you awaken after a dream in the middle of the night, write it down, but try not to turn any lights on in the room.

5. Upon waking in the morning, don't move! Relax your body and think about remembering your dream.

6. Write down whatever you remember right away.

7. If you don't remember anything, try again tomorrow.

JOURNAL ENTRY

Write your dreams from tonight when you wake up tomorrow.

Can you trace them to any events or concerns?

What is your interpretation of your dreams, and did you learn anything from them?

The greatest weapon against stress is our ability to choose one thought over another.

- William James

Until further notice, the days of the week are now Thisday, Thatday, Otherday, Someday, Yesterday and Nextday.

LESSON 30
LESSON: Sense of Touch & Stress

Humans need touch. In the early part of the twentieth century healthy babies in orphanages were dying because they lacked loving human touch. Your skin is your largest organ and has millions of nerve receptors. Touch therapies include hugging people or trees, getting or giving a massage, taking a hot bath or sauna, and petting your dog.

The benefits linked to touch therapies include less depression and anxiety, lower levels of stress hormones, less tension and muscle-skeletal pain, lower and more regular heartbeats, increased alertness, better sleep, and increased immune responses.

Social distancing during the COVID-19 pandemic has left many without their therapeutic hugs which release essential bonding hormones.

One heart-warming solution many have turned to is adopting a pet. In fact, shelters and animal rescue organizations are experiencing a huge surge in adoptions during the pandemic.

So reach out and touch someone – but only if it is safe. If that's not possible, consider adopting a pet you can cuddle with!

Please be responsible about this! Make sure if you adopt a pet you are ready to give it a good home for the duration of its lifetime.

EXERCISE:
Touch and Relax

Touching is important to human development and functioning. Your skin is the largest organ of your body and has one thousand nerve endings per square inch. We are meant to touch and to feel. Do the following to increase your sense of touch (tactile) sensations.

1. Give someone a hug.

2. Give yourself or someone a massage.

3. Rapidly rub your hands and place them over your eyes.

4. Touch nature – flowers, leaves, trees, rocks, and streams.

5. Take off your shoes and walk in the grass or sand.

6. Feel the air temperature and the wind or breeze.

7. There are many, many, many more. Just explore!

JOURNAL ENTRY

Journal how you felt while doing the above touch exercise. What did you touch?

What thoughts did you have while touching the objects?

Did some items make you feel more relaxed?

Did touching help elevate your thoughts and feelings?

Mother Nature speaks in a language understood within the peaceful mind of the sincere observer.

– Radhanath Swami

Having trouble staying at home? Shave your eyebrows off.

LESSON 31
LESSON: Sense of Sight and Stress

Of your five senses, your sense of sight is the most dominant one. As a human race, our sense of sight became highly developed during a time when we didn't have modern cities, televisions, laptops and smart phones, violent movies, 24 hour news, or advertising.

This is important to recognize, because your brain receives and processes millions of signals per second from your sense of sight. You need to be careful what images you allow into your brain for your psychological and physiological health.

Fortunately, the sense of sight can be a powerful tool for relaxation. Viewing images of nature has been proven to decrease tension, lower blood pressure, increase your relaxation response, improve enthusiasm and happiness, decrease mental fatigue, decrease the need for pain medication, and promote health and healing.

You can also relax by closing your eyes and allowing your imagination to wander across the ocean to far off, beautiful lands, or through fond memories with friends and family.

EXERCISE: Color Therapy

Different colors and light affect your mood. Meditate and imagine yourself being surrounded by different colors. Or, if you have the ability, look at colored lights and notice how they affect you. How does each color make you feel?

Red _____

Yellow _____

White _____

Purple _____

Blue _____

Brown _____

Green _____

Pink _____

JOURNAL ENTRY

Find something in nature to watch. Watch a bird or a butterfly, the leaves as they rustle in the wind, or flowers perking up as the sun rises. Observe the life in a stream or a pool of water, watch a bug crawling, or just lie back and watch the clouds in the sky. Take notice of the details.

How does looking at nature affect your mood?

How did you feel before taking time to look at nature? After stopping to look at nature, do you feel less stressed?

The only difference between a diamond and a lump of coal is that the diamond had a little more pressure put on it.

- Anonymous

What do you tell yourself when you wake up late for work and realize you have a fever? Self, I so late.

LESSON 32
LESSON: Sense of Taste and Stress

What we eat and when we eat it affects our emotions, and therefore our levels of stress.

There are certain foods that are proven to increase stress levels, while others help keep stress lower. Foods proven to increase stress levels include greasy foods, alcohol, coffee, and food high in processed sugar. Foods proven to reduce stress include fruits and vegetables, yogurt, and whole grains.

Not only what we eat, but when and how much we eat of any food can add to our stress levels and how we feel about ourselves. Emotional eating is eating to suppress or soothe negative emotions. People sometimes eat when they are stressed, anxious, depressed, angry, fearful, lonely, or bored.

Balance is the key. It's OK to have a small piece of pie or cake at a family gathering, or have a few fries with your meal, just do it in moderation. And try to create an eating plan that mainly includes foods low in sugar and high in nutritional value.

Also, if you are an emotional eater, develop alternate strategies for when you are feeling frustrated, bored, or stressed. Have a plan of action ahead of time, like instead of going to the refrigerator the next time you're stressed or bored, step outside for a few moments to calm your nerves, or dive into a good book or calming app on your phone.

EXERCISE: Eat Away Stress

Choose some of the low-stress foods from the list below. Enjoy the sight of the food, feel the texture, smell it, and then take your time chewing and swallowing. Studies show that you will get more of the food's nutritional value by enjoying it and taking your time eating. Eating is one of the pleasures of life so take time to enjoy it.

Low-Stress Foods

All raw vegetable juices	Carrots, beans, onions
Lettuce, apples, yogurt	Cottage cheese, currants
Raisins, berries, melon	Watermelon, grapes, pears
Peaches, plums, celery, squash	Almonds, brown rice, cabbage
Asparagus, raw spinach, honey	Sesame seeds, millet, rye, oats
Garlic, apple cider, eggplant	

High-Stress Foods

All fried fatty and greasy foods	Alcohol
Beef, veal	Pies, cakes, biscuits
White sugar, white flour	Sardines, tuna
Coffee, tea, cocoa, chocolate	Eggs, gravy, macaroni
Cooking fats, lard	Prepared cereals, crackers

JOURNAL ENTRY

Write about the shape, color, texture, smell, and taste of one of the foods you ate from the above exercise. What were your emotions as you ate the food?

If you are an emotional eater create a plan for what you will do the next time you feel stressed, bored, angry, or sad rather than eating. Write it down here.

Odors have a power of persuasion stronger than that of words, appearances, emotions, or will. The persuasive power of an odor cannot be fended off. It enters into us like breath into our lungs, it fills us up, imbues us totally. There is no remedy for it.

- Patrick Süskind

Due to the panic buying,
Walmart has now opened a 3rd register.

LESSON 33
LESSON: Sense of Smell and Stress

Stress can make your world smell bad. Your sense of smell and your emotions work together. When you are experiencing anxiety you may find you don't enjoy smells that were once pleasant. However, the connection between your sense of smell and emotions can also work in a positive way. There are scents that are proven to reduce your stress and elicit positive emotions.

Think of your favorite cologne, flowers, pine trees, a scented candle burning in your home, or the yummy smell of apple pie. You may also have a scent you associate with a special event or person from your past.

The connection between our sense of smell and our emotions is so powerful there are billion-dollar industries revolving around it, such as the candle and aromatherapy industries. Try it out. Put the following in your bath water or a diffuser and begin to feel the effects.

Stress relief. Chamomile, Lavender, Lemon, Rose, Vanilla, Frankincense

Relieve anger. Chamomile, Jasmine, Rose

Anxiety relief. Cedar wood, Cypress, Lavender, Orange, Frankincense

Increased energy. Peppermint, Cinnamon, Eucalyptus

Improved sleep. Jasmine

Weight loss. Vanilla

EXERCISE:
Aromatherapy

Smells, or aromatherapy, like sights and sounds, can help relieve your stress, improve concentration, increase alpha brain waves, and increase happiness.

What is your favorite smell? Do one of the following to practice aromatherapy for yourself. Also, while enjoying the scents try to take in the sights and sounds associated with them. Listen to the sound of the wind while touching the flower you are smelling, or feeling the grass between your toes. This is how life was meant to be lived, so go enjoy the sights, sounds, and smells of your world as you feel your stress melt away.

- Light a scented candle.
- Crush some peppermint candy and put it in a bowl on the counter in your kitchen.
- Create or buy some potpourri for your home.
- Go to a bath or candle store and smell the different products.
- Go to a health food store and smell the different essential oils.
- Go outside and smell a leaf or flower in your yard.
- Run an orange or lemon peel through your garbage disposal
- Put a dryer sheet in your clothing drawers
- Use an essential oil for a massage, in a burner, or spray it in your home.

JOURNAL ENTRY

Smell items inside your home such as food, candles, and essential oils. Go outside and smell some flowers, trees, and the air around you. Describe how they make you feel.

Do you have any fond memories of a smell from your past, such as your grandma's chocolate chip cookies, the smell on an afternoon spring drive, or a cologne worn by a special person? Write about them.

TODD HUSTON

Sound is the vocabulary of nature.

- Pierre Schaeffer, composer

Day 1 of quarantine:
I'm going to take this as a personal opportunity to improve my health!

Day 2 of quarantine:
Due to personal reasons, I am eating lasagna in my shower.

LESSON 34
LESSON: Sense of Hearing and Stress

Noise, when defined as unwanted sound, is an environmental stressor. The noise does not need to be loud enough to damage your ears. If there is prolonged exposure to an unhealthy noise studies show it can cause sleep disturbances, arterial hypertension, heart disease, and strokes in adults as well as learning and emotional difficulties in children. These noises include aircraft, trains, traffic, loud bars, the buzzing of fluorescent lights, or any noise that is negatively affecting your physical or psychological well-being.

Noise affects you directly through the nervous system and indirectly through your perception, or the way you think about the sound. Both of these pathways have been shown to be associated with stress reactions within your body. The noise may interfere with your daily activities, feelings, and sleep which can make you feel irritable and exhausted, or cause other stress related symptoms.

Sounds can also promote healing and relaxation. Music may inspire you; nature sounds, birds, water, and wind may relax you; or maybe it's the sound of silence you appreciate. Focus on having an environment that promotes your mental and physical health.

EXERCISE:
Nature Sights and Sounds

Numerous studies have shown the benefits of nature in reducing stress. Being in nature can be physically healthy and mentally healing. Sitting quietly and observing nature and listening to its sounds can enhance creativity and promote calm.

Nature has its own music. Though you may not always be able to be outdoors you can still listen to the sounds of nature. Take a moment to listen to the wind, birds, or other animals when you are at work or inside your home. Some of the sounds may inspire you while others calm you. Explore nature and its many sounds.

Enjoyable nature sounds include:

Mountain streams	Humpback whale recordings
Ocean waves	Morning doves cooing
Rainstorms	Ducks
Songbirds	Wind chimes
Waterfalls	Wolves howling
Wilderness sounds	Gentle breeze blowing
Dolphins	Frogs in a pond
Crickets chirping	

JOURNAL ENTRY

Write about a relaxing experience that you had in nature. What did you see and hear that inspired you?

What are some of your favorite nature sounds?

What music relaxes you?

How can you experience the sights and sounds of nature during the Covid-19 pandemic?

The mind is like water. When it's turbulent, it's difficult to see. When it's calm, everything becomes clear.

- Prasad Mahes

Travel plans: trip to the kitchen, then travel to the den for relaxation, a few hikes to the bathroom and then sleep under the ceiling fan in my room.

LESSON 35
LESSON: Mindfulness

Mindfulness consists of paying attention to an experience from moment to moment without drifting into thoughts of the past or concerns about the future. It also includes not getting caught up in thoughts or opinions about whatever situation you currently find yourself in or are hearing about.

Being mindful is important during the COVID-19 pandemic. It will help you relax and overcome fears and anxieties associated with it. Fear is always in the future, so focus on the now.

An easy way to practice mindfulness is through meditation, which involves sitting or lying down quietly. However, you don't have to be lying down to practice mindfulness. You can stop any time during the day, take some deep breaths, and refocus on being in the present.

Focus on being in the NOW!

EXERCISE:
Mindfulness Meditation

Mindful meditation is a mental state achieved by focusing your awareness on the present moment, while calmly acknowledging and accepting your feelings, thoughts, and bodily sensations.

1. Sit or lie quietly and notice your breath moving in and out.

2. Notice anything else you feel in your body.

3. As other thoughts intrude, let them go.

4. Remain aware of being in the present moment.

5. Start to practice for five minutes and then extend to 15 - 20 minutes.

6. As the chatter in your mind settles down you will discover a peaceful state.

JOURNAL ENTRY

Journal your experience during your mindful meditation. Were you able to only think about the present?

What thoughts came to your mind at the beginning, during, and at the end of your meditation?

Did you feel more relaxed and less anxious after meditating? Write some thoughts about your experience.

Yesterday is gone. Tomorrow has yet to come. We have only today. Let us begin.

- Mother Teresa

30 days hath September, April, June, and November, all the rest have 31, except for March which has infinite.

LESSON 36
LESSON: Mental Imagery and Visualization

The images and thoughts you have about the world have been shaped by your parents, friends, and childhood and life experiences. The media and many other external forces also shape your views.

You can change and create your own images of the world. You do not have to accept the images of others, or those you have held on to out of habitual thinking. To create a different and better image for yourself about the world, do the following exercise.

- Hold in thought an image about a specific situation.
- The image must be YOUR image, created by you.
- Think about your image within the context of your values and ideals.
- Surround the image with positive thoughts about yourself, others, and the world.
- Images must be creating a reality that can be real, not a fantasy world.
- Images must be practiced three times per day for 15 minutes each.
- Images must show the process from start to finish.

If everybody practices this, it will not only change each individual's thought, it will change the world, because it will change the way people operate and react to various situations around them.

EXERCISE:
Visualization

This stress tool is effective for healing now and for creating your future. Close your eyes and visualize how you want your life to be one month, one year, five years, and 10 years from today.

Visualize everything about your life. Believe that whatever you want your life to be will come true. Explore what your life would really be like in your image. How do you visualize yourself feeling during each period of time as you successfully accomplish this new life?

There may be some positive changes that have occurred in your life during the COVID-19 pandemic, like more time with family. Visualize any of these changes you'd like to carry forward.

Spend at least 20 minutes doing this relaxation exercise.

Is there anything you would change about your image to make it better?

JOURNAL ENTRY

Journal about the images you visualized in the activity. What did you visualize for yourself? Being strong and healthy? Having a new home in another city? A productive and peaceful life? Your own company? An amazing relationship with your partner? Let your imagination work for you as you create your perfect world in your mind and write about it.

A crust eaten in peace is better than a banquet partaken in anxiety.

- Aesop's Fables

The Coronavirus has achieved what no female has been able to achieve. It has cancelled sports, closed all bars, and kept all guys at home. Ladies, be careful what you wish for!

LESSON 37
LESSON: Resilience

The American Psychological Association (APA) defines resilience as the process of adapting well in the face of adversity, trauma, threats, or significant sources of stress, such as family and relationship problems, serious health problems, or workplace and other stressors. Those with more resilience bounce back better than those with less.

The COVID-19 pandemic has tested people's resilience. Some people feel a greater sense of resilience than others, and this is exhibited in their thoughts, emotions, and behaviors. However, everyone can immediately begin building resilience and spend time building it each day.

Practice these 3 c's to have stronger resilience.

Commitment. Dedication to realizing your full potential within yourself, your family and friends, and your work. You have the ability to overcome the challenge, whatever it is.

Control. A sense of personal control and empowerment in your environment. Though you don't have control over others' thoughts, emotions, and behaviors, you always have control over your own.

Challenge. An ability to see change and problems not as threats, but as opportunities for growth.

Start building your resilience today!

EXERCISE:
Building Resilience

Resilience is a positive adaption to life's stressors.

Think about something you feel has been a stressor in your life. Now think about what knowledge and experience you had to overcome it. You know more than you think about overcoming life's challenges, so dig into your life experiences and think about how you overcame them and how you can apply that knowledge to events and challenges now.

Can you use any of those skills to help you with your challenges during the Covid-19 pandemic?

Build Connections. positive relationships, mentors.

Mind-Body Wellness. healthy diet, exercise, meditate.

Live your purpose. Help others, create goals, explore life.

Stay optimistic. Be hopeful, look for the good in everything and everyone.

JOURNAL ENTRY

Write about a difficult experience in your past. Write about what happened and how you felt. Also write details about it, like what you were wearing or where you were.

Take a moment to write about positive things that have come from that experience. Maybe it's something you learned that made you stronger. Maybe it's a skill you learned that has helped you since then. Maybe you realized you are a survivor who can overcome anything. Write about it.

Practice random kindness and senseless acts of beauty.

- Ann Herbert

Nurse: Your coronavirus test came back positive.
Me: That can't be correct! I have more than 300 rolls of toilet paper!

LESSON 38
LESSON: Social Support

Social support from family, friends, co-workers, and others can help minimize the effects of stress, boost the immune system, and add quality to your life.

Face to face interaction is best. Being with someone in person allows you to get the full benefits of social interaction. This has not been easy during the COVID-19 pandemic. People are having to remain socially distanced while talking to family, friends, and neighbors. Facetime, Facebook Live, What's App, Zoom, and other video chat platforms have provided great solutions for this, giving people the opportunity to reach out and see their friends and loved ones while staying at home.

Texting is the least preferred option because it does not allow face-to-face interaction. Studies show that people who text lose their ability to communicate as well as those who use audio or visual means of communication. They don't always pick up on verbal and non-verbal cues as well as those who have more face-to-face interactions.

Whatever form of communication you choose, USE IT! Even if you feel stressed or depressed and don't feel like reaching out, call someone you trust and share what you're going through. Also take time to discuss enjoyable things about your day. You typically find it lifts your spirits and helps you move forward on a more positive path.

EXERCISE:
Support Therapy

Spend time today with a friend, family member, loved one, or another supportive person in your life. Also, offer them support, especially if they are struggling with a challenge at work, home, or within themselves.

Work together to come up with solutions. If that's not possible, simply be there to offer a loving, listening ear. Take some time during the conversation to talk about something positive as well, to help deescalate stressed or depressed emotions.

Another idea is to do something kind for someone and ask for nothing in return. Try to do it without them knowing if you can.

Using these ideas provides you with more opportunities to decrease your stress levels. Though people appreciate your concern and help, research on unconditional love actually shows that the helper feels a greater emotional benefit from helping others than those they are helping feel.

JOURNAL ENTRY

Write about a conversation you've had with someone where you helped them out with a challenge they were facing. What emotions did you feel while you were talking to them?

How did you feel during and after the conversation? Did they appreciate your support?

What did you learn about yourself?

A good laugh overcomes more difficulties and dissipates more dark clouds than any other one thing.

- Laura Ingalls Wilder

They said that a mask and gloves were enough to go to the supermarket. They lied, everyone else has clothes on.

LESSON 39
LESSON: Humor

Laughter is the best medicine. There's a good reason for that popular saying. Humor helps people feel better immediately, but can provide long-term relief for mental and physical ailments. When using the correct type of humor, it is great for stress reduction. Try feeling stressed while laughing. Not easy to do, is it?

There are four types of humor.

Affiliative humor. This is psychologically healthy humor and can lower the stress levels for everyone in a stressful situation. It decreases tension and improves relationships while allowing people the space to look at the situation in a different and more positive way. Jerry Seinfeld or James Corden.

Self-enhancing humor. This is good natured humor and the ability to laugh at yourself or your situation. You find a way to take something that may be perceived as negative and make it funny. Ellen DeGeneres

Aggressive humor. This style of humor is sarcasm and ridicule. The constant put-downs are hurtful to everyone's mental health, including the jokester. It often involves prejudices. You may laugh but it is at the expense of another, which doesn't bring you any real sense of joy. Chelsea Handler, Daniel Tosh, comedy roasts

Self-defeating humor. This humor has the jokester putting themselves down with disparaging humor. Putting yourself down in an aggressive or "poor me" fashion is called self-defeating humor. This type of humor can lead to lower self-esteem and increased levels of stress. Rodney Dangerfield.

Affiliative humor and self-enhancing humor help reduce stress and depressive symptoms, while increasing optimism and psychological well-being. It is more psychologically healthy than aggressive or self-defeating styles of humor.

EXERCISE:
Laugh Away Your Stress

Humor can decrease stress. Laughter stimulates the body's organs by increasing oxygen intake to the heart, lungs, and muscles, and lowers blood pressure. With the pandemic our world is currently facing, it's important to note that laughter increases immune cells and infection-fighting antibodies that help fight disease. This is obviously a positive thing, especially during the COVID-19 pandemic.

Do you feel stressed? Find an Instagram account, funny movie, television show, or book that uses positive styles of humor, such as affiliative or self-enhancing humor. Many people enjoy funny videos or memes with animals. There are great Instagram accounts out there with hilarious satirical humor that doesn't aim to hurt or bash. Notice how your mood and thoughts change about your stress after you begin watching.

JOURNAL ENTRY

Think about your mood before, during, and after looking at, or watching, something funny. Did you notice having a better mood while you were doing this? Maybe it helped you feel more optimistic or come up with a creative solution to a problem you are dealing with. Write about it.

Think of something stressful in your life. See if you can come up with a joke about the situation, or write something funny about it. Write it out and see if it helps reduce your stress about the situation.

Never forget the three powerful resources you always have available to you: love, prayer, and forgiveness.

- H. Jackson Brown, Jr.

I don't know why my fishing buddy is worried about Coronavirus, he never catches anything.

LESSON 40
LESSON: Forgiveness

Psychologists generally define forgiveness as a conscious, deliberate decision to release feelings of resentment toward a person who has harmed you. Forgiveness does not mean condoning or excusing the offense.

Forgiveness frees you from negative emotions, such as hurt and anger, and allows you to feel at peace. The stressor may be caused by another person, or by your own actions, but you are the one who feels the weight of unforgiveness.

For forgiveness to be effective, it must be *unconditional*. Only then does it break the connection between your negative emotions and your feelings of unforgiveness. The Journal of Behavioral Medicine found there are medical conditions tied to practicing *conditional* unforgiveness which can cause early death. This means you can't say, "I will forgive you *if* you say you were wrong," or, "I will forgive you *if* you promise to do better." You can work with the other person to create solutions to the problem, but this is separate from forgiveness and letting go of your resentment and anger.

Benefits associated with forgiveness include lower stress levels, improved mental health, more positive emotions, a stronger immune system, improved heart health, and higher self-esteem.

Learn to let go to let yourself live!

EXERCISE:
Nine Steps to Forgiveness

Dr. Luskin of Stanford University conducted the Stanford University Forgiveness Projects. From this, *Nine Steps to Forgiveness* was developed, which is a simple and effective guide to improving your ability to forgive.

Step 1. Know exactly how you feel about what happened and be able to articulate what about the situation is not OK.

Step 2. Make a commitment to yourself to feel better.

Step 3. Forgiveness does not necessarily mean reconciling with the person who upset you or condoning the action.

Step 4. Get the right perspective on what is happening.

Step 5. At the moment you feel upset, practice stress management to soothe your body's fight, flight, or freeze response.

Step 6. Give up expecting things from your life or from other people that they do not choose to give you.

Step 7. Put your energy into looking for another way to get your positive goals met than through the experience that has hurt you.

Step 8. Remember that a life well lived is your best revenge.

Step 9. Amend the way you look at your past so you remind yourself of your heroic choice to forgive.

JOURNAL ENTRY

Unsent Letters

Write a letter to your boss, spouse, friend, or someone you feel has hurt or angered you. DO NOT send it - throw it away. You are simply writing about it to help you work through your emotions.

Now write a forgiveness letter and throw it away. Tell the person you forgive them. Also write about forgiving yourself for carrying hurtful thoughts toward them. Those feelings are normal – everyone feels them. YOU are working to let them go, which is what matters.

Think about how you behave toward someone you have not unconditionally forgiven and write about it. Be honest with yourself.

Gratitude turns what we have into enough.

– Anonymous

My body has absorbed so much soap and disinfectant lately, now when I pee I clean the toilet.

LESSON 41
LESSON: Gratitude

Gratitude is the act of being thankful. You may feel gratitude toward someone who has been kind, supportive, or helpful, such as your partner, a friend, a stranger who smiles unexpectedly at you, or God. It can also be an emotion you feel for nature, your newly decorated home, or your new bicycle you are excited to start riding. Gratitude helps you connect to something outside of yourself, making it a positive experience for all involved.

Gratitude has been shown to increase your mental well-being; decrease feelings of isolation, loneliness, and stress; boost your immune system; help with sleep; increase your joy and happiness; and strengthen your social and business relationships. Everyone appreciates being appreciated.

You may have to practice saying thank you because it may feel awkward at first, but it will quickly become a habit and you will immediately begin to feel the benefits.

EXERCISE:
Gratitude in Action

Here are some ways Harvard University Medical School recommends to express your gratitude.

Write a thank-you note. You can make yourself happier, and nurture your relationship with another person, by writing a thank-you letter expressing your enjoyment and appreciation of that person's impact on your life. Also, occasionally write a thank you note to yourself.

Thank someone mentally. Send a thank you note with your positive thoughts toward someone you appreciate.

Keep a gratitude journal. These are available on-line and at bookstores. They vary so be sure to get one that matches your needs and personality.

Count your blessings. At the end of each day, think about positive things that happened and how it impacted you. Even if it was a "bad" day, look for something you can be grateful for. If you look hard enough, you will find something.

Pray. Prayer means different things to everyone. It can be taking time to get quiet and becoming open to something outside of yourself that is caring for you. Or it can be simply shutting your eyes and quietly recognizing the good that is going on.

Meditate. Focus on the present moment and what you are grateful for in your life right now.

JOURNAL ENTRY

Write about what you are thankful for in your life.

What is something you are grateful for today?

What is something you are grateful for from your past?

List several people you appreciate being in your life. Write a note, call, or have video chat with one of them to say thank you.

How has saying "thank you" made you feel?

Does this path have a heart? If it does, the path is good; if it doesn't, it is of no use.

- Carlos Castaneda

During self-isolation.

Dogs: "Oh my gosh! You're here all day and this is the best as I can love you, see you, be with you and follow you! I am so excited because you are the greatest and I love you being here so much!"

Cats: "Why are you still here and how long until you leave?"

LESSON 42
LESSON: Love

Love is the greatest power this world has ever known and everyone possesses its strength. With it you can change yourself and the world. Love is the international language. Studies show when people are more loving they feel more at peace and live longer. But what is love?

I love chocolate, I love my partner, or I love football. Love has been defined many ways. Music, movies, advertisers, and the media make love even more confusing. Billions of dollars are spent every year trying to convince you of a product or service that will bring love into your life. However, love is never found externally. It is always found internally. This power that will change you and the world is always within you everywhere you go.

Who taught you love? Your parents or caregivers? A special teacher who saw your potential? A preacher at your place of worship? Hopefully their expression of love was unconditional. Unfortunately, that isn't always the case. Unconditional love has no fear, shame, or guilt associated with it. When you love others, or yourself, with unconditional love, you love only to love. No conditions.

The COVID-19 pandemic has brought more unconditional love out of people. People are selflessly serving others, often with no reward. Live with unconditional love toward all, and you will find greater peace and health in your life.

EXERCISE:
Life is a Lesson in Love

Love is the most important lesson to learn in life. You will learn your lessons about love with people you love as well as those you don't, and many you will never know. Every place, every person, and every situation is teaching you a lesson of love if you are willing to learn it. Do you have a family member who lovingly tells you "good morning" every day, no matter how you acted the day before? Or did some random person smile at you, even though you were frowning? They are each teaching you about unconditional love. Is there a coworker who is driving you crazy, and you have to dig deep to be more patient? They are helping you go within to learn more about unconditional love. Did you have to learn to control your temper because you didn't want to unleash it on your children? They came into your life to help you learn more about unconditional love. Ever watched a mother bird hovering over her baby on a stormy day? What a great example of unconditional love!

There is no chance encounter. You can try to avoid the lessons of love but you can't postpone them. The lesson will eventually find another way to reach you. Though these lessons are sometimes tough, they are to your advantage. The more you learn and know love, the happier you will be.

When is the best time to learn love?

The answer is always the same, now! Go out there today with this in mind, and see what lessons of love come your way.

JOURNAL ENTRY

What is your definition of unconditional love?

When was the first time you felt pure and unconditional love? Was it in nature? While praying? Or was it something someone said or did for you?

How are you living unconditional love in your life?

What opportunities did you have to learn love today?

One song can change a moment, one idea can change a world, one step can start a journey, but a prayer can change the impossible.

- Anonymous

So many coronavirus jokes out there, it's a pundemic.

LESSON 43
LESSON: Spirituality

Many people find their spiritual beliefs comfort, inspire, and give them hope in times of stress. They feel their spiritual beliefs and practices can overcome many, if not all, of life's challenges. Stressors can compel a person to begin a spiritual journey. Stressors can also strengthen spiritual beliefs that have proven helpful in the past.

There are four processes to nurturing spiritual growth while decreasing stress.

1. **Centering.** Reflect on who you are and your purpose in life. Get still and quiet. Listen for your inner voice.

2. **Emptying.** Recognize negative thoughts are normal, and don't condemn yourself for having them. Let them sit quietly next to you, or imagine them floating gently away down a river. Replace them with loving thoughts about yourself, others, and your Higher Power.

3. **Grounding.** Grow into your spirituality. Explore new ideas and knowledge to enhance your spiritual growth.

4. **Connecting.** Recognize the relationship of *one* with the *whole*. You are not alone, and you are loved. You are connected to all of life and to your Higher Power.

EXERCISE:
Prayer

Prayer has been scientifically proven to work. It can lower anxiety, increase optimism, and instill hope. The act of prayer is different for everyone. For some people it is taking time to get quiet and meditate, while to others it is a religious exercise. Regardless of what form your prayer takes, the following guidelines from prayer researchers have been suggested to make it more effective.

1. Find a quiet spot and clear your mind.

2. Pray in present tense and believe your prayers will work.

3. Phrase your prayers in a positive manner. Avoid words such as *can't* and *don't*. For example, say "I am healthy," or, "I'm praying about health," rather than, "I must not get sick."

Spend some time in prayer today. Don't forget to add all the things you are thankful for, or to recognize and pray about those who might be needing your prayers right now.

JOURNAL ENTRY

Write about your spiritual beliefs and how they benefit you in your life.

How are your spiritual beliefs helping you during the COVID-19 pandemic?

What spiritual questions would you like answered?

Write about a prayer that has been meaningful to you.

The day she let go of the things that were weighing her down, was the day she began to shine the brightest.

- Katrina Mayer

I think this quarantine is making people a little crazy. This morning I saw a neighbor talking to her cat. It was obvious she thought her cat understood her. I came into the house, told my dog...we laughed a lot.

LESSON 44
LESSON: Maintaining Your Stress-Resilient Life

Congratulations! You have completed the Mental Survival Guide, COVID-19 Edition. You now have within your possession an incredible arsenal of tools to help you feel empowered over stress. The COVID-19 pandemic will pass, but you will likely come across other stressful situations in the future. By going through this course and its activities, you have begun to develop some stress-resilient habits. Practice them! Watch for situations that trigger you to feel stress so you are prepared to react to them in a more positive, healthy way. By doing this, you take away the power of stress. It will no longer be that silent monster that has been draining your life or roaring at you and disrupting your peace.

Think back to which stress tools worked best for you. When you find yourself in a stressful situation use it! Take a moment to think about what you can do to deescalate the situation internally and externally. You will likely be surprised by how much more seldom stress shows up in your life, and when it does, how quickly it leaves you.

Above all, these tools will help you create the life that you want – full of peace, love, joy, meaning, and fun.

EXERCISE: Relaxation Reminders

To remind you to practice the relaxation exercises in this book each day, place sticky notes in your home, office, or car, or set alarms on your phone. Maybe it's to remind yourself to breathe deeply, set aside some time to meditate, or check out a funny video or meme. Maybe you want to periodically do a One Minute Body Scan to see if you are clenching your jaws or feel tension in your shoulders. Did you start a gratitude list? Remind yourself to add to it. Do you know someone who needs some encouragement? Shoot them a text or give them a quick call to let them know you're thinking of them. Review your SMART Goals, or time management worksheets to make sure you're staying on track. Did stepping out into nature for a couple of moments relax you? Do you find comfort in prayer? Does taking a 10 minute break to get some exercise help relieve stress?

Whatever it is that works for you, take the time to do it! You are worth it! Your feelings of peace and joy are worth it! Not only will it help you be better for others, more importantly you will be better for yourself.

JOURNAL ENTRY

Which stress management tools did you find most helpful?

List which techniques you will use, how often, and when.

Enjoy the new opportunities for love and peace while living a life with reduced stress. Write about the positive changes you see taking place in your life by doing this.

LOGS
Anger Log

Example

Situation: My wife didn't cook dinner tonight

Thoughts: She doesn't appreciate me or my hard work

Feelings: Angry, depressed

Physical Response: Fast breathing and heart, face got red

Actions: Slammed the door, yelled at her

Outcome: She started crying, told me she was going to her mom's

Next time: Will call wife and cook together, bring food home, or dine out. Ask her about her day, maybe it was stressful for her too.

Your Turn

Situation:

Thoughts:

Feelings:

Physical Response:

Actions:

Outcome:

Next time:

LOGS
Goal Log

I, _____, am going to _____
   (your name)   *(activity or goal)*

for or by _____. I will measure my goal
          (how long, how often, by when)

by _____ every _____ and
   (method to measure progress towards goal)   *(how often)*

be accountable to _____. When I have completed
                  (person's name)

this contract, I will reward myself by _____.
                                       (something that motivates you)

LOGS
Sleep Log

Date _____

How was your overall energy and mood yesterday before going to sleep?
_____

What did you do to relax before going to bed?
_____

What time did you get into bed? _____

How long did it take you to fall asleep? _____

How many times did you wake during the night? _____

How many hours did you actually sleep? _____

What time did you wake this morning? How did you feel?

_____

How was your overall energy after you woke up today?
_____

Did you have any of the following today? Nap, caffeine drinks, alcohol, exercise?
_____

What was your overall stress level on a scale from 1-10, with 1 being low and 10 high? _____

TODD HUSTON

Eisenhower Matrix
Urgent-Important Matrix

Do
Tasks you will do immediately

Ex: Project Planning

Schedule
Tasks you will schedule to do later

Ex: Health checkup, Exercise

IMPORTANT | **URGENT** | **NOT URGENT** | **NOT IMPORTANT**

Delegate
Tasks you will spend less time with and delegate to someone else

Ex: Replying to certain emails

Eliminate
Tasks that you will eliminate

Ex: Web Surfing, Watching TV

LOGS
Time Management Skills

URGENT / IMPORTANT

Deadlines, Exams, Real Emergencies, Important Meetings

MANAGE

NOT URGENT / IMPORTANT

Planning, Problem Prevention

FOCUS

URGENT/NOT IMPORTANT

Some calls and emails, Most Drama

AVOID

NOT URGENT/NOT IMPORTANT

Social Media, Facebook, Twitter, Instagram

LIMIT

Worksheet

My to-do list to categorize in Urgent/Important Table

# Begin to work on tasks in the following order.

URGENT / IMPORTANT

_____
_____
_____
_____
_____
_____
_____

NOT URGENT / IMPORTANT

_____
_____
_____
_____
_____
_____
_____

Begin to work on tasks in the following order.

URGENT/NOT IMPORTANT

_____
_____
_____
_____
_____
_____
_____

NOT URGENT/NOT IMPORTANT

_____
_____
_____
_____
_____
_____
_____

Stress Tests
How Susceptible Are You to a Stress Related Illness

Life Stress Test
By Dr. Tim Lowenstein

In the past 12 months, which of the following major life events have taken place in you life?

1. Make a check mark next to each event that you have experienced this year.

2. When you're done, add up the points for each event.

3. Check your score for susceptibility to stress-related illness

_____ Death of spouse 100
_____ Divorce 73
_____ Marital separation 65
_____ Jail term 63
_____ Death of close family member 63
_____ Personal injury or illness 53
_____ Marriage 50
_____ Fired from work 47
_____ Marital reconciliation 45
_____ Retirement 45
_____ Change in family member's health 44
_____ Pregnancy 40
_____ Sex difficulties 39
_____ Addition to family 39
_____ Business readjustment 39
_____ Change in financial status 38
_____ Death of close friend 37
_____ Change to a different line of work 36

_____ Change in number of marital arguments 35
_____ Mortgage or loan over $10,000 31
_____ Foreclosure of mortgage or loan 30
_____ Change in work responsibilities 29
_____ Trouble with in-laws 29
_____ Outstanding personal achievement 28
_____ Spouse begins or stops work 26
_____ Starting or finishing school 26
_____ Change in living conditions 25
_____ Revision of personal habits 24
_____ Trouble with boss 23
_____ Change in work hours/conditions 20
_____ Change in residence 20
_____ Change in schools 20
_____ Change in recreational habits 19
_____ Change in church activities 19
_____ Change in social activities 18
_____ Mortgage or loan under $10,000 17
_____ Change in sleeping habits 16
_____ Change in number of family gatherings 15
_____ Change in eating habits 15
_____ Vacation 13
_____ Christmas season 12
_____ Minor violations of the law 11

_____ **Your Total Score**

SCORING SHEET

_____ **0-149** Low susceptibility to stress-related illness.

_____ **150-299** Medium susceptibility to stress-related illness. Learn and practice relaxation and stress management skills and a healthy lifestyle.

_____ **300 and Over** High susceptibility to stress-related illness. Daily practice of relaxation skills is very important for your wellness. Take care of it now before a serious illness erupts or an affliction becomes worse.

NOTE: This scale shows the kind of life pressure you are facing. Depending on your coping skills or lack thereof, this scale can predict the likelihood of you falling victim to a stress-related illness. The illness could be mild (frequent tension headaches, acid indigestion, and loss of sleep) or very serious (ulcers, cancer, migraine, heart problems, etc.)

What You May Experience If You Have Stress

1. Frequent headaches, jaw clenching, or pain
2. Gritting, grinding teeth
3. Stuttering or stammering
4. Tremors, trembling of lips, hands
5. Neck ache, back pain, muscle spasms
6. Light-headedness, faintness, dizziness
7. Ringing, buzzing, or "popping" sounds
8. Frequent blushing, sweating
9. Cold or sweaty hands, feet
10. Dry mouth, problems swallowing
11. Frequent colds, infections, herpes sores
12. Rashes, itching, hives, goose bumps
13. Unexplained or frequent "allergy" attacks
14. Heartburn, stomach pain, nausea
15. Excess belching, flatulence
16. Constipation, diarrhea, loss of control
17. Difficulty breathing, frequent sighing
18. Sudden attacks of life-threatening panic
19. Chest pain, palpitations, rapid pulse

20. Frequent urination

21. Diminished sexual desire or performance

22. Excess anxiety, worry, guilt, nervousness

23. Increased anger, frustration, hostility

24. Depression, frequent or wild mood swings

25. Increased or decreased appetite

26. Insomnia, nightmares, disturbing dreams

27. Difficulty concentrating, racing thoughts

28. Trouble learning new information

29. Forgetfulness, disorganization, confusion

30. Difficulty in making decisions

31. Feeling overloaded or overwhelmed

32. Frequent crying spells or suicidal thoughts

33. Feelings of loneliness or worthlessness

34. Little interest in appearance, punctuality

35. Nervous habits, fidgeting, feet tapping

36. Increased frustration, irritability, edginess

37. Overreaction to petty annoyances

38. Increased number of minor accidents

39. Obsessive or compulsive behavior

40. Reduced work efficiency or productivity

41. Lies or excuses to cover up poor work

42. Rapid or mumbled speech

43. Excessive defensiveness or suspiciousness

44. Problems in communication, sharing

45. Social withdrawal and isolation

46. Constant tiredness, weakness, fatigue

47. Frequent use of over-the-counter drugs

48. Weight gain or loss without diet change

49. Increased smoking, alcohol, or drug use

50. Excessive gambling or impulse buying

Lesson 12: Values and Goals
JOURNAL ENTRY Selection (page 63)

- Accountability
- Accuracy
- Achievement
- Adventurousness
- Altruism
- Ambition
- Assertiveness
- Balance
- Being the best
- Belonging
- Boldness
- Calmness
- Carefulness
- Challenge
- Cheerfulness
- Clear-mindedness
- Commitment
- Community
- Compassion
- Competitiveness
- Consistency
- Contentment
- Continuous Improvement
- Contribution
- Control
- Cooperation
- Correctness
- Courtesy
- Creativity
- Curiosity
- Decisiveness
- Democraticness
- Dependability
- Determination
- Devoutness
- Diligence
- Discipline
- Discretion
- Diversity
- Dynamism
- Economy
- Effectiveness
- Efficiency
- Elegance
- Empathy
- Enjoyment
- Enthusiasm
- Equality
- Excellence
- Excitement
- Expertise
- Exploration

- Expressiveness
- Fairness
- Faith
- Family-Orientedness
- Fidelity
- Fitness
- Fluency
- Focus
- Freedom
- Fun
- Generosity
- Goodness
- Grace
- Growth
- Happiness
- Hard Work
- Health
- Helping Society
- Holiness
- Honesty
- Honor
- Humility
- Independence
- Ingenuity
- Inner Harmony
- Inquisitiveness
- insightfulness
- Intelligence
- Intellectual Status
- Intuition
- Irreverence
- Joy
- Justice
- Leadership
- Legacy
- Love
- Loyalty
- Making a difference
- Mastery
- Merit
- Obedience
- Openness
- Order
- Originality
- Patriotism
- Perfection
- Piety
- Positivity
- Practicality
- Preparedness
- Professionalism
- Prudence
- quality relationship
- Reliability
- Resourcefulness
- Restraint
- Results-Oriented
- Rigor
- Security
- Self-actualization

- Self-control
- Selflessness
- Self-reliance
- Sensitivity
- Serenity
- Service
- Shrewdness
- Simplicity
- Soundness
- Speed
- Spontaneity
- Stability
- Strategic
- Strength
- Structure
- Success
- Support
- Teamwork
- Temperance
- Thankfulness
- Thoroughness
- Thoughtfulness
- Timeliness
- Tolerance
- Traditionalism
- Trustworthiness
- Truth-seeking
- Understanding
- Uniqueness
- Unity
- Usefulness
- Vision
- Vitality

Common Thought Distortions Begin to work on tasks in the following order. that May Increase Stress

What are thought distortions?

Instant and automatic thoughts about yourself, others, or life.

Other names.

Irrational thoughts, Automatic thoughts, Dysfunctional thoughts, Cognitive distortions, Pessimistic self-talk.

What do they do?

Distort reality and contribute to feelings of anxiety, stress, depression, anger, helplessness, distrust, hopelessness, or fear.

How do I change them?

Become aware of, and change, any distorted thoughts by challenging and modifying them.

- Recognize the stressful situation or event.
- Identify your uncomfortable mood or feelings.
- Identify what your body is feeling (headache, tightness, etc.)
- Identify the thinking distortion.
- Challenge it to see if it measures up to objective evidence.
- Choose and use an alternative response.

Our thoughts make stressful events worse

The following are common types of unproductive and distorted stress-produced thinking.

Childlike Fantasy. Assuming, as children do, that everything should go your way.

"Everyone should be nice and love one another."

Deep Mistrust. Expecting that others willfully mistrust, dislike, manipulate, or take advantage of you.

"Others are just out there to get me."

Negative Fortune Telling. Consistently predicting the future negatively, typically thinking that things will never change or only get worse.

"I'll never get money or be content with life."

Needless Perfectionism. Having a virtually impossible standard for yourself.

"It is all my responsibility and I should not make mistakes."

Helplessness. Believing you can't do anything for yourself and must have help from others.

"I can't deal with anything on my own."

Imperfections/Feelings = Unlovability. Thoughts that you are basically defective and flawed, which makes you unlovable by others if they found out.

"If anyone finds out I'm not as good as I pretend to be they will not accept me."

Catastrophizing. Turning simple frustrations, irritations, and disappointments into unbearable disasters and catastrophes.

"I didn't get the job so my world is over."

Special Privilege. Feeling like you have a special privilege or entitlement or that you deserve more respect and attention than you get.

"I should always get what I want because I deserve it."

Task Exaggeration. Treating simple barriers or challenges as overwhelming or insurmountable.

"If I don't see a solution, why even try it."

Unrealistic Isolation. Feeling that you are different and isolated from the rest of the world.

"I don't belong. I am too different and no one understands me."

Possibilities = Probabilities. Thinking that if it is possible for something to go wrong, then it probably will.

"If it can go wrong, I will mess it up."

Musts, Oughts, and Shoulds. Turning simple honest desires, wants, and expectations into absolute musts, oughts, and shoulds.

"I must be successful or famous!" "I ought to have that dream or perfect boyfriend." "I should be able to get into that Ivy League college."

VS

"It would be cool to be successful or famous." "It would be great to get my dream job or have an awesome boyfriend." "I'm going to work hard to get into that Ivy League college."

Rigid, Either/Or Thinking. Viewing events or people in all-or-nothing, right-or-wrong terms, and not considering "shades of gray."

"It feels like no one can be trusted."

Needless Other Blaming. Looking for someone else to blame when things don't go right.

"It's my wife's fault I always feel bad."

Unrealistic Need for Love and Approval. Having a need for love and approval that is so strong it influences what you say and do with others.

"I must always get people to love and accept me."

Negative Spin. Arbitrarily and pessimistically putting a negative interpretation on events, even though they may be neutral or positive.

"My life is always bad and things never turn out like I want them to."

Emotion-Distorted Thinking. Letting your negative feelings color and distort how you see the facts.

"I feel depressed and nothing seems right."

Ignoring Contrary Evidence. Focusing on negative evidence while ignoring or discounting equally relevant positive evidence.

"No one likes me. I will never succeed."

Needless Self Blame. Making a problem worse by needlessly blaming yourself for negative events, shortcomings, or imperfections; failing to see that some events have other, complex causes.

"My relationship is so bad and it is all my fault."

Regretting the Past. Focusing on past problems rather than what you have or can do now. Believing you cannot impact the future due to past events.

"My life has been filled with so many failures that I can do little about the future."

Minimizing/Avoiding. Understanding or avoiding the true significance of events resulting in problems eventually becoming worse than inaction.

"Things will get better on their own."

Mind Reading. Believing you know what others want, think, or feel without asking.

"He doesn't like me." "I know what he wants."

What If? What If? What If? Constant asking "What is?" something happens, and failing to be satisfied with any of the answers.

"I can't do that! What if I get scared?"

Fatalism. Believing that the uncontrollable powers of fate determine the present, and there is little you can do about it.

"No use in trying to make things better; it's going to be bad anyway."

Comparing Worth. Thinking you are not "as good as" someone else in all areas.

"Why can't I have what he has, then people would like me."

Resources for Mental Help Assistance During Covid Pandemic (USA)

National Hotlines for the COVID-19 Pandemic

911 for emergency

CDC.gov

Disaster Distress Helpline, call 1-800-985-5990, or text TalkWithUs to 66746

Substance Abuse and Mental Health Services Administration Disaster Distress Helpline: 1-800-985-5990 or text TalkWithUs to 66746

National Suicide Prevention Hotline 1-800-273-8255

National Domestic Violence Hotline or call 1-800-799-7233 and TTY 1-80-787-3224

National Child Abuse Hotline: 1-800-4-A-CHILD (1-800-422-4453) or text 1-800-422-4453

https://preventchildabuse.org/coronavirus-resources/

https://www.caregiver.org/coronavirus-covid-19-resources-and-articles-family-caregivers

For Healthcare Professionals and Organizations

https://www.ama-assn.org/delivering-care/public-health/caring-our-caregivers-during-covid-19

https://www.ama-assn.org/system/files/2020-04/caring-for-health-care-workers-covid-19.pdf

Internet search the following for your location

Search for your local mental health hotlines

Search for local food pantries and shelters

Search for local mental health specialists, psychiatrists, psychologists, psychotherapists, social workers, and other mental health care providers.

https://www.stress.org/

About Todd Huston M.A.

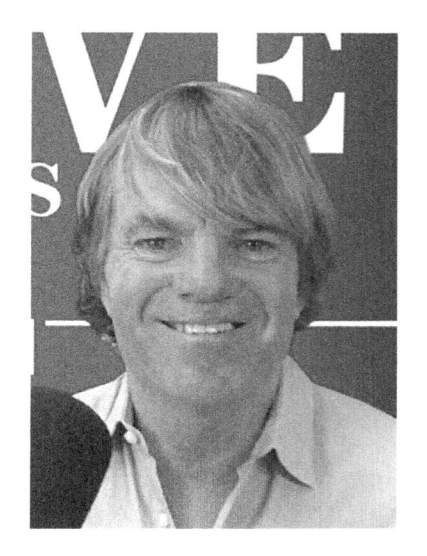

Todd Huston knows how to overcome incredible challenges and overwhelming stress in life. When his legs got caught in the propeller of a boat at age 14, his life was radically changed. He battled to keep his legs with numerous surgeries, but the bone disease eventually forced him to have one leg amputated.

Todd became a psychotherapist in California. He also worked in psychiatric hospitals for adults, adolescents, and children. He used his professional skills and personal experiences to help patients achieve more in their lives. He also led workshops training health-care professionals, corporate executives, Fortune 500 companies, mental health clients about stress management and techniques.

Todd has done the unimaginable. To prove that anyone can overcome challenges he completed a world-record-setting Summit America expedition by climbing to the highest elevations of all 50 states in only 66 days 22 hours and 47 minutes, shattering the original record by 35 days!

Todd has been featured in thousands of publications throughout the world, including Sports Illustrated, Forbes, and the Wall Street Journal, and popular books such as Chicken Soup for the Soul, A Second Helping.

He has appeared as a special guest on CBS Year in Sports and Robert Schuller's Hour of Power. Todd has been interviewed on ABC, NBC,

CBS, CNN, TNN, Inside Edition, Extra, plus numerous radio programs.

Todd is the host of Love Leaders Podcast. Where he interviews experts and inspiring individuals

Several distinguished honors have been awarded to Todd including U.S. Jaycees' Ten Outstanding Young Americans (President John F. Kennedy and Gerald Ford, Elvis Presley, Peyton Manning) the Henry Iba Award for Outstanding Citizen Athlete (Carl Malone, Nancy Kerrigan), the Class Act Award, The Power to Dream Achiever Award, American Red Cross's Everyday Hero Award and the Distinguished Eagle Award (Neil Armstrong, Steven Spielberg, Nobel winners)

About Julie Dunbar, LMSW

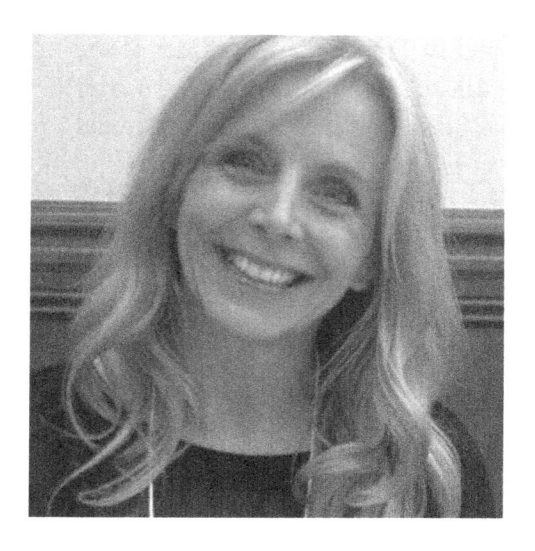

Julie Dunbar, LMSW is a full-time psychotherapist and life coach. She loves working with families, children and couples. She is a certified high-ropes course instructor where she teaches youth, adults, business and community leaders confidence building and team building skills. She loves the outdoors and enjoys running, biking, competing in triathlons and mountain climbing. Her first priority is "being a mom" to her five children and dog "Z". She is known for her bright smile, cheerfulness and wisdom.

ENDORSEMENTS

Being a psychologist in New York City, I'm on the front lines of the COVID-19 mental health pandemic. The symptoms and casualties of stress are obvious everywhere. Todd's book, COVID-19 Mental Survival Guide, gives everyone great tools they can use now to overcome the emotional and mental challenges everyone is facing during these times and when life returns to normal. Read this book and regain your peace of mind.

Mark Borg, Jr., PhD
Author: Irrelationship: How We Use Dysfunctional Relationships to Hide from Intimacy

∽

Navy SEALS taught me to be tough in battle and Todd taught me how to be tough in life. Read his book, COVID-19 Mental Survival Guide so you can win the mental battle during this pandemic.

Mike Bay
U.S. Navy SEAL Team 5, ret.

∽

Todd has written this masterpiece in order to help those who are in need of a feel-better and/or start-over. The skills in this book could help anyone overcome a struggle that might be experienced during their own personalized pandemic situation.

Samantha Cannon LCSW, EMDR

ENDORSEMENTS

Are you looking for a comprehensive stress management program specifically designed to help you excel in these uncertain COVID-19 times? If so, look no further. Todd Huston weaves a tapestry of personal and professional expertise to create a tangible survival guide in 44 digestible lessons. Whether you are a first time learner or seasoned health care professional, Todd's handbook will become a priceless life survival guide to be used for years to come.

Debra A Stone LCSW, APRN

Around 70% of adults say they feel stress or anxiety daily. Stress wreaks havoc on our physical health, emotional equilibrium, and mental health. While it may seem like there's nothing you can do, the Mental Survival Guide book is an incredible resource full of education, tools, and practical resources to help you relieve stress and make healthy changes in your life.

Jordan Green LCSW

NOTES

NOTES

NOTES

NOTES